PMS HELL TO PMS HARMONY

EMMA LOUISE KIRKHAM

Copyright © 2022 by Emma Louise Kirkham

All rights reserved. This book or any portion thereof may not be reproduced or used in any manner whatsoever without the express written permission of the author except for the use of brief quotations in a book review.

First Published 24th June 2022
Last updated: 30th October 2022

Disclaimer

All information contained within this book is for informational purposes only. It is not intended to diagnose, treat, cure or prevent health problems – nor is it intended to replace the advice of a qualified medical practitioner. Always consult your physician or qualified health professional on any matters regarding your health or on any opinions expressed within this book.

The information provided within this book is believed to be accurate based on the best judgment of the author, but the reader is responsible for consulting with his or her own health professional on any matters raised within. We do not assume liability for the information contained within this program, be it direct, indirect, consequential, special, exemplary, or other damages.

It is always advisable to consult your physician before changing your diet, starting an exercise program, or taking supplements of any kind, especially if you have pre-existing medical conditions. Also, in relation to any suspected conditions you may be seeking to address, you should always consult a doctor for any relevant testing requirements to either confirm or rule out your suspicions.

Table of Contents

DISCLAIMER ....- 3 -
INTRODUCTION ....- 7 -
   Who This Book Is For ....- 10 -
   Who This Book Is NOT For ....- 11 -
GETTING STARTED ....- 13 -
PART 1: THE LOWDOWN ON PMS ....- 15 -
   Introduction to Your Menstrual Cycle ....- 17 -
   Seed Cycling for your Menstrual Cycle ....- 27 -
   That Week Before ....- 35 -
   The Symptoms of PMS ....- 38 -
   The causes of PMS ....- 41 -
PART 2: EXCESS ESTROGEN ....- 45 -
   What is High Estrogen? ....- 47 -
   The Causes of High Estrogen ....- 49 -
   Raising Progesterone ....- 51 -
   Beware the Estrogen Imitators ....- 55 -
   Why Weight Matters ....- 62 -
   Feed Your Flora ....- 69 -
   Look After Your Liver ....- 74 -
PART 3: GLUCOSE INTOLERANCE ....- 81 -
   What is Glucose Intolerance? ....- 83 -
   Let's Talk Sugar ....- 89 -
   Balance Blood Sugars Through Diet ....- 93 -
   Reduce Inflammation ....- 101 -
   Stress Less ....- 105 -
   Sleep Yourself Healthy ....- 111 -
   Exercise or Excess Insulin ....- 117 -
PART 4: VITAMINS & MINERALS ....- 121 -
   How vitamins and mineral deficiencies impact on your PMS ....- 123 -
   Essential Fatty Acids ....- 126 -
   Vitamin B6 ....- 130 -
   Vitamin D ....- 132 -

ZINC	- 135 -
CALCIUM	- 138 -
MAGNESIUM	- 141 -
SUPPORT YOUR PMS WITH NUTRITION	- 144 -

PART 5: MOVING INTO PMS HARMONY ....- 145 -

KEEP GOING	- 147 -
RESOURCES	- 149 -
NEED ADDITIONAL SUPPORT?	- 151 -

REFERENCES ....- 153 -

ABOUT THE AUTHOR ....- 157 -

Introduction

I first began my periods when I was ten years old. I remember waking up one morning to find my bedding covered in blood and the most goddamn awful cramps in my stomach. Instinctively, I knew what was going on despite never having had "the talk" from my parents. I walked into my parents' bedroom and calmly announced to my mother, who was still in bed, what had occurred only to be given money and told to go to the shop to buy myself some pads from the corner shop.

As a child, I was teased horribly for my early puberty. I was an early developer in all aspects and at 9 years old I was getting my first bra. Now, when most young girls were going getting crop top style starter bras or AA cups, I began my bra life in an A-cup after nagging my mum that I needed one. Maybe she wanted to deny the fact I was developing, which is why it took so long for me to convince her that I needed one!

Something else I remember from childhood, was crying in pain when those period cramps occurred. The bleeding was often so heavy it would go through onto my clothing. It was so bad that I would have to take the day off school and spend the day curled up in a ball with a hot water bottle pressed firmly against my abdomen and taking two paracetamol every four hours, wishing the burning, stabbing sensation would end. I never really grew out of that stage, I just traded the paracetamol and hot water bottle for codeine and anything else I could get my hands on. Yet as a child, I don't really remember having PMS.

As I got older though, things seemed to get worse. In the week before my period I'd be short tempered, snappy and irritable, go through bouts of feeling down or anxious, get breakouts of spots around my jawline and generally feel like I couldn't be arsed with anything or anyone. Then suddenly a week later my period would arrive and I'd be "Ahhhh … that's why I've been a total bitch".

For over 30 years I have struggled with my periods, with the only respite to the heavy bleeding and crippling cramps happening when I was pregnant or when I had the Mirena coil fitted (which only truly worked the first-time round).

Despite many visits to the doctors and having tried several differing contraceptives and the various medications I was prescribed, which probably did more harm than good for my estrogen levels, nothing shifted those feelings and reactions. I became resigned to the fact this was how life was going to be, a week or two of being a bitch followed by 2-3 days of horrific pain, nausea and heavy bleeding when my period did arrive.

It was only when I reached 40, a couple of years ago, that I decided I wanted to stop filling my body with imitation hormones and instead try to follow a more natural approach towards my health and wellbeing. As part of that, I had my Mirena coil removed, despite the warnings from the gynecologist that I would likely get back the severe cramps and want it back in.

She was right, they came back with an absolute vengeance, and my PMS also seemed to be worse than before too (which I later discovered is an actual thing, the older you get, the worse your PMS gets if it's left unchecked).

So, after completing my health coach training, I decided to specialise in hormone health, undergoing further training and going on my own personal journey of hormone healing. I wanted to understand my body and find ways to make Mother Nature's monthly visit more bearable. It's an ongoing journey for me, because hormones are forever … not just for PMS week!

This is what led me to create this book. My mission is to help the many women out there who suffer unnecessarily on a monthly basis with their menstrual cycle and their PMS hell, including you.

Because that's why you're here right? You've been reading along and nodding your head at some of the things I describe suffering from, because it resonates with you, because you experience them too, and because you want to find a way to make it more bearable for yourself and for those who have to put up with you when you're like a snarling beast.

But before we get started let me clear up a couple of things:

Who This Book Is For

This booked is for you lovely, yet fed-up, ladies who are struggling to manage with your PMS and who are ready to start making changes RIGHT NOW.

Perhaps you're fed up of riding the rollercoaster of emotional ups and downs, you're feeling kind of bad for making your partner or your families lives hell once a month, or you're sick to death of feeling like you can't function when those PMS blues kick in.

It's for those of you who want to discover why this is happening to you, to understand the causes behind it all, and to discover steps you can take to regain control over those raging hormones. It's for those of you who are willing to make lifelong changes in order to restore your mental and physical health throughout your menstrual cycle which is going to take place every week of every month. There's no escaping it, well … until menopause kicks in but even then, that opens a whole new can of worms!

It doesn't matter if your PMS symptoms are mild or severe, the advice given in this book will help you to restore balance when it comes to your pre-period struggles. The fact you've purchased and started reading this book, means the intention to get started is there but, before you do, let me give you a reality check as to what to expect by reading the next section on who this book is NOT for.

Who This Book Is NOT For

This book is most definitely NOT for those of you who are looking for a quick fix and who are not willing to make sacrifices and changes. If that sounds like you, then put this down right now and go find some fluff and nonsense book that makes those false promises of quick fixes and happy ever after.

When it comes to regaining control over raging hormones, you have to be prepared to make a long-term commitment to looking after your mind and body through nutritional and lifestyle changes. Yes, some of my clients have started to notice improvements after only a few weeks but I advise everyone to commit to at least three months, especially when introducing supplements into your lifestyle as it takes three months to start seeing real results from supplements. You'll actually notice in this revised edition, I've put the Vitamins and Minerals part of the book at the front instead of the end as this should be one of your first starting points.

I can give you the advice and the tips but, at the end of the day, it's down to you to implement those changes and in my experience, you have to truly want to change things. If you're half on the bench and half off it, you won't succeed as you'll get bored and give up. That will leave you feeling deflated. You'll give yourself false belief that the methods don't work but at the end of the day, it's because you didn't follow it through.

Harsh, but true! So, the question now is …

Are you ready to get started on a journey that will take you from PMS hell to PMS harmony?

Getting Started

You have invested in me and my book, and I want you to get the very best results from the advice I have to share. So, to help get your journey off to a great start let me give you a few pointers:

Download Your Workbook

I've created a handy and downloadable workbook for you to use alongside this book. It includes a menstrual cycle tracker, meal planner, shopping list, goal setting worksheet, and more. The workbook will give you three months of planning and journaling to help support you on your journey from PMS Hell to PMS Harmony. Get your copy from my website **www.emmalouisekirkham.com** for 50% off when you enter the code WORKBOOK at the checkout.

Keep an Open Mind

Before you go any further into this book … be sure you are truly ready to make changes. You need to go into this with an open mind, to be ready to experiment with new ideas and foods and to be prepared to cut back (or even get rid of) the things that do not serve you or your hormones anymore. It's time to spice things up …quite literally!

Make Sure You've Got Support

It's always easier to achieve your goals if you've got support around you. Don't be afraid to tell friends and family about what you are doing and why, that way it's going to be easier for you to make the changes and, you never know, they might even take part with you. You can even reach out to me via my **Instagram** DMs or tag me **@emmalouisekirkham** to share your goals, achievements and keep yourself accountable. Let me be your cheerleader too!

Remember You are in Control

Yep, I said it. You ARE in control, despite what you might think. You hold the power in your own hands to heal yourself and your PMS. I can give you the tools and the advice, but it's down to you to implement it. So, if you really want to regain control over your PMS and you are raring to go, grab yourself a cuppa (I'd recommend a nice cup of herbal tea, not coffee, as coffee can disrupt your hormones), get yourself comfortable and let's begin …

Part 1: The Lowdown on PMS

Introduction to Your Menstrual Cycle

When looking at our PMS, it's all related to the hormonal changes that take place throughout our menstrual cycle (and a few other factors that we will be looking at throughout this book), so the best place to begin is by reacquainting yourself with your menstrual cycle.

I know I might be telling you things you already know, but when it comes to our menstrual cycle we tend to just accept it as one of those things that just happens on a monthly basis. We forget to remind ourselves of what is going on during each stage of our cycle and how to best care for ourselves during each stage, so that's what we are going to look at now.

The menstrual cycle is broken down into four phases; the follicular phase, the ovulatory phase, the luteal phase and the bleeding (or menstruating) phase. Although PMS generally takes place in the luteal phase, it's worth having an understanding of what takes place during each phase and what is a normal cycle.

Generally, a 'normal' cycle can be anywhere from 25-35 days. Anything less or more than this range should be checked out by a doctor as it can be an indication of an underlying condition. Better to be safe than sorry, right?

Follicular phase

This phase tends to begin the first day of your period and ends the day before ovulation. Often described as the 'spring' of our menstrual cycle, its corresponding moon phase is the waxing moon. During this phase the ovaries are getting the egg prepared and ripened, and there are several hormonal changes taking place in the body (luckily these changes tend to have a more positive effect).

At the beginning of the follicular phase your levels of estrogen and testosterone are low but they do tend to rise slowly throughout this phase helping to boost your energy levels, your mood, your confidence and your brain skills. This makes you feel more confident, more vibrant and more alive.

The rising testosterone will stimulate your libido meaning your other half could be in for a treat, ooh la-la, whilst rising estrogen improves the condition of your skin and hair and pushes you to want to be more social.

As ovulation draws closer the uterine lining begins the thicken, the cervix which has been in a lower position and closed, will gradually start to open and you'll notice your cervical fluids (aka discharge ... who actually thought of that word as it's not the nicest!) will start to become wetter as that estrogen builds up and may start to look creamy in the days before ovulation.

Behind the scenes during this phase, the pituitary gland will release follicle stimulating hormone (FSH) which stimulates the follicles that the eggs are stored in causing (usually) one of them to mature. The pituitary gland will then release luteinising hormone (LH) to stimulate ovulation.

Follicular Phase Best Practices:

- Starting new projects at work or at home
- Making important decisions (both business and/or personal)
- Problem solving
- Strategy building
- Getting out and about to socialise with others
- High intensity exercise and strenuous activities

Follicular Phase Foods:

During the follicular phase you want to be eating foods that help support oestrogen function, including:

- Pumpkin seeds
- Flax seeds
- Pomegranates
- Sprouted beans
- Avocados
- Coconut or grass-fed butter

Ovulatory Phase

The ovulatory phase is a pretty short one lasting only 2-3 days. Often described as the 'summer' of our menstrual cycle, its corresponding moon phase is the full moon. This is the phase when the egg is released from the ovary and begins its journey down the fallopian tube and into the uterus, should it become fertilised.

Just before ovulation the body produces a surge of luteinising hormone which causes the follicle holding the egg to burst. The egg then has around 12-24 hours for it to become fertilised. If it doesn't it will simply disintegrate. This is why ladies who want to get pregnant should be getting their jiggy on a few days BEFORE ovulation, as sperm has a better lifespan and can last for up to 5 days in the fallopian tubes.

During this phase our cervix moves up higher meaning any sperm attempting to fertilise the egg have further to swim. Although it sounds a bit harsh, this is to ensure that only the best quality sperm make the journey … interesting how our bodies dictate natural selection! You'll also notice that cervical fluids are generally clear, sticky and stretchy, a bit like an egg white. This is a huge sign you are 'fertile' however some women may just have very wet and watery cervical fluids, and that's totally normal too. Remember, we are all unique so all you need to do is learn what is normal for you, not everyone else.

Hormone wise, your estrogen and testosterone are at their peak which means you're likely to feel like Samantha from Sex and the City! Your sex drive is at its highest, you're looking and feeling at your most attractive and everything in your body is quite literally screaming "I'm fertile, take me now!"

Ovulatory Phase Best Practices:

- Anything task or activity where you need to be on your 'A game'
- Job interviews
- Highly important conversations (you know, the ones you put off)
- Networking and public speaking events
- Launching a new business or product
- Scheduling a date night
- Any type of physical exercise, activity or sport

Ovulatory Phase Foods:

During the ovulatory phase you want to eat foods that support liver detoxification as this will prevent oestrogen dominance when levels are at their peak. These foods include:

- Flaxseeds
- Brussel sprouts
- Kale

- Cabbage
- Turnips
- Broccoli

Luteal Phase

You've been enjoying the wave of feeling amazing, then here comes the luteal phase to really screw you over as this is the phase where your PMS is going to kick in if the egg is not fertilised.

This phase is sometimes described as the 'autumn' of our menstrual cycle, its corresponding moon phase is the waning moon. This is probably also the longest phase of the menstrual cycle, lasting around 12-16 days and it is split into two parts.

During the first half of the luteal phase, you'll start by having a rapid drop in FSH and LH levels, these will stay low for the rest of your cycle. Estrogen and testosterone levels also become lower but progesterone levels rise as the follicle that released the egg transforms into a temporary endocrine that produces progesterone called a 'Corpus Luteum'.

This causes our body temperature to rise slightly (which if you do go on to track your menstrual cycle, which I talk about later, you should notice) making us like a mini incubator for the egg in preparation for pregnancy.

This rise in progesterone also stimulates the growth of the uterine lining, again as the body prepares for a fertilised egg to be implanted and will change our cervical fluids from that wet and stretchy phase to being stickier and drier. There is no nice way to talk about vaginal fluids, so bear with me on this!

During this time, it's often described as the 'nesting phase' ... you know, where momma bird starts preparing the nest. So, we tend to want to be more organised during this phase and we also tend to have a keener eye for detail.

Then comes the second half of the luteal phase, where estrogen levels rise slightly to finish preparing the uterine lining for pregnancy, but when that doesn't happen our state of being organised and in control of our sh*t goes well and truly out of the window.

Estrogen and progesterone levels will drop rapidly causing the onset of our PMS and the uterine lining to shed during the next phase (our actual period). This sudden drop in hormone levels is notoriously difficult for so many women, causing that range of physical and/or emotional symptoms that we will be looking at as we move further into this part of the book.

Luteal Phase Best Practices:

- Clearing your social calendar, you'll be much more content at home!
- Practicing self-care: massages, baths, etc
- Indulging in a little chocolate, but make sure it's dark chocolate with at least 80% cocoa content
- Enjoy healthy and nourishing comfort foods, like soups and stews
- Gentle exercise like yoga
- Getting that extra hour or two of sleep

Luteal Phase Foods:

During the luteal phase you want to eat foods that support progesterone production and those that are high in vitamin C and vitamin B6. These foods include:

- Oranges
- Peppers
- Grapefruit
- Bananas
- Walnuts
- Salmon

Menstruating Phase

Also known as the bleeding phase, I can assure you that, for me, it is most definitely no bleeding fun either. The menstruating phase is often referred to as the "winter" of our cycle, its corresponding moon phase is the new moon.

The uterus lining that was being broken down at the end of our luteal phase is now being shed and, in conjunction with some muscle contractions, it is expelled from the body as our period.

Our periods can vary in length, 4-5 days is classed as 'optimal' but they can range from 2 to 7 days. Blood should start out a healthy red colour (a bit like the colour of cranberry juice), some people may have blood clots, but as everyone is slightly different the key is identifying what's normal for you (which is another great reason for tracking your menstrual cycle which we are looking at next).

It's definitely a time for a lot of self-love and, believe it or not, some physical touch, as orgasms release oxytocin which can help reduce the physical pain of our period. I don't know about how your period impacts on you but, I know I certainly do not feel in the mood for a tumble in the bedsheets when my period arrives, but never say never right!

Menstruating Phase Best Practices

- Journaling, goal setting, and creating vision boards
- Self-love and self-care, including those hot, relaxing baths
- Very gentle exercise such as yoga
- Self-massage & hot water bottles (especially if you suffer cramps)
- Physical touch (it releases oxytocin which can reduce physical pain!)

Menstruating Phase Foods

During this phase you want to be including foods that are rich in minerals, vitamins and iron, to replenish what the body loses when bleeding. These foods include:

- Mineral rich bone broth
- Vitamin rich smoothies
- Comforting soups and stews
- Beans and legumes
- Leafy green vegetables
- Liver & animal protein

Seed Cycling for your Menstrual Cycle

Seed cycling is becoming all the rage, I hear it mentioned all the time on social media.

The theory behind seed cycling is that consuming different seeds at different stages of your cycle can help boost hormone levels and, is believed to reduce many of those PMS symptoms we experience.

The four seeds used in seed cycling are flax, pumpkin, sesame and sunflower seeds. The reason these are alternated throughout your cycle are because of the different oils, vitamins and minerals they supply and how they can either help stimulate the production or assist in the detoxification of oestrogen and, also help with the metabolism of both oestrogen and progesterone – the two main hormones involved in your menstrual cycle.

Here's how seed cycling works:

During your menstruating and your follicular phases, you should be consuming flaxseeds and pumpkin seeds.

Flaxseeds help balance our estrogen levels by raising it as needed, due to their phytoestrogenic properties, but also by helping remove excess estrogen from the body due to the lignans they contain. Plus, flaxseeds are a great source of fibre which helps keep you feeling fuller for longer and helps your body remove waste products.

Pumpkin seeds contain high levels of zinc which helps support progesterone production in the luteal phase. By consuming them in the first half of your cycle you are helping your body prepare for the second half.

During your ovulatory and luteal phases, you should be consuming sesame seeds and sunflower seeds.

Sesame seeds can help alleviate cramps and help boost immunity as they are a rich source of magnesium and calcium. They are also high in lignans, which means they help support oestrogen balance, and are a good source of omega-6, which helps to support progesterone levels and help fight inflammation.

Sunflower seeds are also high in omega-6. They also contain magnesium and are rich in selenium, which helps support the liver as it removes not only waste products in general, but excess estrogen from the body.

You can add seeds to yogurt, smoothies, salads, soups, stir fries, and baked goods just to give you a few ideas of how to incorporate them into your diet.

Tracking Your Menstrual Cycle

I always advise my clients to track their menstrual cycles on a daily basis. There are several reasons for this:

- **You get to learn what is a 'normal' cycle for you.** We are all unique and different in the length of our cycle, and in the duration and flow of our period. By tracking your cycle, you learn what your 'normal' is, which gives you a baseline to work from and identify when things may me going awry.

- **It helps to track when you're fertile.** For my clients who are trying to get pregnant, tracking basal temperature and cervical fluids can help them identify when they may be at their most fertile and plan for that sexy night in for two.

- **You can easily spot changes.** By knowing what your baseline 'normal' is, you can easily identify when something isn't quite right.

- **It can be presented to your doctor.** There may be times when you need to visit a doctor due to menstrual cycle irregularities. Tracking your cycle means you can present your doctor with a month on month account of EXACTLY what is going on with your cycle which can help support any concerns you may have.

So, for all the reasons given above, I'm going to advise you to track yours too! I've created a handy tracking sheet that you can use which will help you look at changes during all the stages of your cycle including cervical fluids, menstrual fluids, physical and emotional changes so you can learn more about how your body responds throughout the different stages of your cycle. You'll find three tracking sheets in the supporting workbook if you have purchased this, alternatively one is in this book for your reference.

Let me guide you through the things you will be checking for when tracking your cycle:

Tracking your Cycle Length

Firstly, it's good to identify the length of your cycle. This can be beneficial as it can help you identify if you have any issues with length or timings of your cycle. If the cycle is 24 days or less in length, this may indicate you have luteal phase defect (which can be caused by low progesterone or stress), or if the cycle is more that 35 days in length this may indicate issues such as PCOS, excess estrogen, peri-menopause or premature ovarian failure.

Equally, they say the 'healthy' and optimal length of a period is 4-5 days, but if your period is 7 days and it's always been 7 days, then that's your normal and you don't need to strive to fit the medical textbook definitions.

Tracking Your Cervical Fluids

Tracking your cervical fluids (a.k.a. your vaginal discharge) can help identify the different stages of your cycle and help identify when you may be at your most fertile. Again, I know it's not the most pleasant thing to be paying close attention to but it can easily help you spot any changes, or issues such as possible infections. When we looked at the stages of the menstrual cycle earlier, I talked about how cervical fluids may be during those different stages so if you need to refresh your memory, just flick back to that section.

Tracking your Menstrual Fluids

Another less appealing, but incredibly useful thing to track is your menstrual fluids during your period (a.k.a. the blood during your actual period). Tracking the flow and consistency of menstrual fluids can help identify possible hormonal imbalances. If you have heavy bleeding, clots or lumpy blood, this can indicate that estrogen levels are high, whereas if the blood is more pink and thinner in consistency it could actually indicate low levels of estrogen. That information in itself is useful, as it means you will become aware whether you need to look at ways to balance your oestrogen and progesterone.

Physical and Emotional Symptoms

Tracking both physical and emotional symptoms helps to identify how you feel at certain times of your cycle. Being aware of these changes can help you plan for them (or forewarn your loved ones of the approaching whirlwind of emotions about to begin!). For instance, you know that for a certain number of days during your cycle you are prone to feeling depressed; as these days approach, you are able to plan in lots of self-care activities, and clear out your social calendar.

Body Temperature

Tracking your body temperature is more commonly heard of in women who are trying to get pregnant. That's because it can help you to identify if you've ovulated. In fact, the body temperature can change by 0.3 – 0.7 degrees after ovulation as the body prepares to 'incubate' a fertilised egg, however, by the time you notice these changes there's little point getting down and dirty with the other half, as the egg is likely to be deteriorating already.

So why do I want you to track your body temperature? Because, that rise in temperature tells you that you've ovulated, meaning you know exactly what stage of your cycle you are at (and obviously you can thank me later if this nugget of wisdom helps you create a mini version of you at a later date).

So, as you can hopefully see, identifying what is a normal menstrual cycle for you gives you that baseline to work from and can help give you early warning signs as to anything being wrong. An example would be, if your period was always 7 days in length but suddenly started being 2-3 days in length ... that's an indication you should go get checked by the doctor as that's not 'normal' for you.

To help with your menstrual cycle tracking, as I mentioned earlier, I've created a tracking chart for you to use. You can find it in your workbook so, be sure you've downloaded and printed off a copy so you can start tracking right away, alternatively you'll find a copy of it on the next page.

Menstrual Cycle Tracker

		1	2	3	4	5	6	7	8	9	10	11	12	13	14	15	16	17	18	19	20	21	22	23	24	25	26	27	28	29	30	31
Temp	Temperature (if tracking)																															
Physical Symptoms	Nausea or Vomiting																															
	Cramps																															
	Sore/Tender Breasts																															
	Headache/Migraine																															
	Bloated																															
	Tired																															
Emotional Symptoms	Tense and on edge																															
	Depressed																															
	Forgetful																															
	Confused																															
	Anxious																															
	Irritable / Easily Annoyed																															
	Happy																															
Blood Colour	Brown																															
	Red																															
	Pink																															
Menstrual Fluids	Bleeding - Clotting																															
	Bleeding - Heavy																															
	Bleeding - Normal																															
	Bleeding - Light																															
	Bleeding - Spotting																															
Cervical Fluids	Cloudy/Milky																															
	Creamy																															
	Thick																															
	Watery																															
	Sticky																															
	Clear																															
	Dry																															
	Day	1	2	3	4	5	6	7	8	9	10	11	12	13	14	15	16	17	18	19	20	21	22	23	24	25	26	27	28	29	30	31

Month: Jan / Feb / Mar / Apr / May / Jun / Jul / Aug / Sep / Oct / Nov / Dec

That Week Before ...

We know it well, we come to anticipate it. Our partners dread it and quite often know we are there way before we do as they catch the razor-sharp slash of our tongues when our shorter than usual temper kicks in, or because we turn into a blubbering mess for no apparent reason over the slightest thing they say or do.

There have been many times I've been grumpy and grouchy but unable to put my finger on why. Then one morning, I wake up and my period has arrived. That's when the realisation occurs that it was my PMS and I have to make my mumbled apologies to those who were caught in the hormonal tornado only days before.

In fact, the things us women can do during our period can be both hysterically funny or downright terrifying. Women have shared stories of throwing their partners dinner out after some flippant comment was made, screaming obscenities at items of cutlery, bursting into tears because their dogs looked at them funny, and others have admitted to throwing objects at their poor unsuspecting partners.

In fact, coming to think of it ... I think I once threw either a cup or a plate at my ex-husbands head once because he said something that obviously didn't go down too well with me. Whoops, my bad! But FYI, that's not the reason he's my ex-husband.

But, by far the best PMS story I came across was the woman who flew from London to Canada after an argument with her boyfriend. Yep, that's right ... she literally grabbed a bag, stormed out of the house to Heathrow airport and flew to her aunts in Toronto. That was one expensive bout of PMS, I'm sure.

But all joking aside, PMS is far more than just being a bit of a moody cow that week before our period arrives (in fact, some women can have PMS for 3 out of 4 weeks). There's a whole range of unwanted side effects we get and, both the severity and symptoms can vary from person to person.

If we start by looking at what PMS is, it is a term used to describe the physical and emotional symptoms that many women experience in the latter part of their menstrual cycle. In other words, the symptoms we often experience in the week running up to our actual period however, these symptoms can actually appear at any time in our cycle and can last three to five days after our period begins - thanks for that one Mother Nature!

The definition 'many women' that is commonly used is also rather vague. In fact, it is believed that over 90% of women experience some form of premenstrual symptoms. These symptoms can range from mild to severe, and approximately one third of women who suffer with painful periods have pain that is so severe they need to miss work or school.

It's also common for PMS to get worse as you get older, especially as you approach peri-menopause and menopause due to decreasing hormone levels.

It's really no joking matter, especially if you are the one suffering it, but luckily help is at hand in the form of this book.

The Symptoms of PMS

The symptoms of PMS are probably familiar to you, especially if you're reading this book - you're here to learn how to regain control over it, right? So, do forgive me if I'm repeating things that you already know.

What may surprise you the most when it comes to PMS symptoms, is that there are over 150 physical, emotional and behavioural symptoms have been associated to PMS … WOW!!!!

However, the ones that are commonly referred to and the ones you are most likely to experience are:

- Mood swings
- Fatigue
- Bloating
- Abdominal cramps
- Irritability
- Breast Tenderness
- Depression
- Anxiety
- Headaches or Migraines
- Brain Fog
- Spotty skin (especially around your jawline)
- Greasy hair

Oh yep, it's a barrel of fun isn't it. We feel like crap and then, to really stick the knife in, we look like crap too with spotty skin and scraped back greasy hair ... but that's just those of us who have it 'easy' as there is a far darker and less spoken about side to PMS.

For some women, their PMS symptoms can be much, much worse to the point it can cause major disruption to their day to day life. In addition to the symptoms we looked at above, women may also experience additional symptoms such as:

- Feelings of sadness, hopelessness or worthlessness
- Decreased interest in your usual activities
- Difficulty concentrating even on simple task
- Tension, anger, and increased conflict in relationships
- Insomnia or excessive sleeping
- Feelings of being overwhelmed

When this happens, it's often referred to as PMDD (Pre-Menstrual Dysphoric Disorder). PMDD is actually a serious, chronic condition that is often mistaken for chronic depression as the symptoms associated to the two conditions are very similar. PMDD is believed to affect 3% - 8% of menstruating women and it can be so bad that some women who suffer with it have reported feeling suicidal.

I've often seen lists of PMS symptoms stating that some of these PMDD symptoms are a 'normal' part of PMS. Let me tell you ladies, it's really not 'normal' to feel that way! There is NOTHING 'normal' about that, no matter what anyone tells you!

What I find even worse, is that women who do get diagnosed with PMS or PMDD are often given pharmaceutical medicines to boost serotonin (think anti-depressants) and/or oral contraceptives ... but are we just masking the problem when we do this? Or even aggravating the problem, as pharmaceutical medicines can often disrupt our gut lining which can then cause further issues with our hormones, throwing our hormones out of whack and having a domino effect on how our PMS effects our life.

Now don't get me wrong, I'm not saying pharmaceutical medicines cannot help, nor am I suggesting you stop taking any medications you have been prescribed. But, as these issues root back to hormonal imbalances, I believe we can help support our bodies and improve our symptoms by making dietary and lifestyle changes. After all, that's what this book is about and that's what I'm here to help you with.

The causes of PMS

So, we know what PMS is and we know the symptoms, but what actually causes PMS in the first place?

Although research has yet to define the exact causes of PMS, throughout our menstrual cycle we go through various hormonal changes, including changing levels of estrogen and progesterone which are key players in our PMS symptoms appearing.

PMS will generally occur in the luteal phase of your menstrual cycle. The luteal phase begins just after ovulation and typically lasts around 12-16 days. In the initial stages, the body is preparing for pregnancy. levels of estrogen and testosterone drop and levels of progesterone increase to allow the thickening of the uterine lining so that the egg, if fertilised, can embed itself there.

During the second week of this phase, estrogen levels begin to rise again in order to support the preparation of the uterine lining for pregnancy. When pregnancy does not occur (which is a relief for some of us and a curse for others) then levels of both estrogen and progesterone drop massively which means 'hello' to feeling like crap and triggers the PMS.

These fluctuations of our hormone levels also have an influence on the chemicals in our brain that control our levels of serotonin, dopamine and oxytocin - also known as our mood hormones. This does explain why we go through so many mood swings as women (it's all about the science ladies, not that we are crazy lunatics) and it's also why we often crave chocolate around our period, as chocolate has been well documented as being a mood boosting food due to triggering the same mood-based chemical reactions in our brain.

So hopefully you've now got a better idea of the hormonal fluctuations that impact on your menstrual cycle and how they relate to your PMS. Now, let's take a look at the three key areas that can cause PMS symptoms to be worse for some than others. These are:

1) Estrogen Dominance
2) Glucose Intolerance
3) Vitamin and Mineral Deficiencies

Each of these areas of imbalance are influenced by their own set of potential causes. Over the course of this book I'm going to be looking at each of these areas in more detail with you and I will be giving you all the advice you need to start taking your PMS from a state of PMS hell to PMS harmony.

It's completely your choice which area you want to begin with, as I've designed the rest of this book so you can pick and choose which area you want to work on first. However, when I'm working with my one-to-one clients I generally advise them to start supplementing from the beginning as it will take up to three months for supplements to start showing results.

My advice for you, as you move forwards on your journey, is to choose two to three lifestyle or dietary changes from the section you are working on and really focus on these for the next two weeks. Once they become a part of your regular routine, add in another 2-3. Spend around 4-6 weeks on each subject (i.e. estrogen dominance) to give yourself the best possible results.

Don't rush onto the next section until you've fully implemented the steps of the previous section and it's become a regular habit. Small and lasting changes along the way will lead to better results than trying to do everything at once and failing. Rome wasn't built in a day, nor was hormone balance.

Part 2: Excess Estrogen

What is High Estrogen?

Our hormones have an effect on every cell and tissue in the body however, some have more of an impact than others on our menstrual cycle and, in particularly, on our PMS symptoms.

Oestrogen is our primary hormone as a woman. It's mainly produced in our ovaries, but it can also be produced by the adrenal glands and, in our fat cells. It's our levels of estrogen that are responsible for our womanly shape, the size of our boobs and the size of our butts. It also plays a role in our vaginal lubrication which is why many women experience vaginal dryness as they approach and hit menopause.

Estrogen is often believed to be just one hormone and I get why, it's so often spoken about as being one entity, but in reality, there are around 15 different types of estrogen. The three main types of estrogen associated to a woman's menstrual cycle are Estradiol (E2), Estrone (E1), and Estriol (E3).

The estrogen that's linked to our PMS is estradiol (E2). It's the form of estrogen that's the most common in women of reproductive age and the type of estrogen that facilitates your menstrual cycle and the release of your eggs during ovulation. It also has benefits for the heart, bones, brain and colon, but hey, we are here for the PMS right, so let's not let me get off track!

High levels of estrogen in the body is known as estrogen dominance and it can cause havoc with our menstrual cycle. When you look at some of the symptoms of high estrogen it includes things like breast tenderness and cysts, PMS, fibroids, endometriosis, menstrual migraines, irritability, moodiness and frequent meltdowns (hell, yes to those!), depression and weepiness, and midcycle ovulatory pain. It has also been linked to breast and ovarian cancer.

Wow, that's one hell of a nasty list when it comes to being a woman right? So, you can see that many of these signs of estrogen dominance are also the symptoms that we experience when we have PMS.

To be able to tackle our PMS and regain control over those raging hormones we do need to address excess levels of estrogen in the body and that's what we will be doing in this part of the book as we move on to looking at the causes of high estrogen and then looking at the individual ways of tackling them.

The Causes of High Estrogen

High oestrogen, or oestrogen dominance as it's also known, is a multi-system issue. That means there are several factors in the endocrine system that play a role in its development.

The main causes of high estrogen tend to be high cortisol levels, caused by stress on the mind or body, low progesterone levels, xenestrogens, which are fake estrogens that come from our environment and personal care products, excess body fat and, excessive alcohol consumption. Gut imbalances, blood sugar imbalances and thyroid problems can also play a role.

Estrogen dominance has a major impact on our menstrual cycle as it prevents the brain from sending out follicle stimulating hormone (FSH) and luteinising hormone (LH) which is what induces follicle maturation and ovulation. Due to this, it can be a major problem for ladies who are trying to get pregnant.

Did you also know that high estrogen can also dramatically reduce your sex drive? High levels of estrogen can block the body from producing testosterone, and low levels of testosterone can cause a decreased sex drive. So, if you've not been feeling in the mood for a little rough and tumble in the sheets lately, high oestrogen could be to blame.

Throughout this section of the book, I'll be covering some of the main causes of high estrogen for you to address in your life. These include, raising progesterone levels to bring estrogen back into balance, spotting and avoiding the infiltration of sneaky estrogen mimickers, how your weight impacts on estrogen levels, looking after your gut flora, and helping your liver dispose of excess estrogen.

As with anything in this book, choose one area to focus on for a week or two. Once you've got that mastered and it becomes a habit, move on to adding in the next stage. Remember, it's not a race or a quick fix, it's about making lifelong changes that will support you through your PMS struggles and beyond.

Raising Progesterone

Progesterone works alongside our oestrogen and aims to keep everything in perfect balance. It's our keep calm and carry on hormone, having an effect on our mood, sleep, nervous system and helping to ease anxiety.

However, it is primarily produced during the second half of the menstrual cycle, you know, the phase where our beloved PMS kicks in! During this latter part of our cycle, a temporary endocrine gland in the ovary, known as the corpus luteus, produces progesterone in preparation of pregnancy. It helps prepare the uterus lining, thickening the walls, so the fertilised egg can transplant itself into it where it will develop and grow. If pregnancy doesn't occur, levels drop, as I mentioned when we looked at the stages of the menstrual cycle.

Estrogen dominance occurs when estrogen and progesterone levels are out of balance, and there is more estrogen in the body than there is progesterone. As these two hormones work hand-in-hand, you cannot have high oestrogen without having low progesterone.

PMS or PMDD are just one of the signs of low progesterone, causing symptoms such as disrupted sleep, low moods and anxiety. Other symptoms are quite similar to those of high estrogen and include menstrual migraines, heavy bleeding during your period, irregular menstrual cycles, swollen or painful breasts, and spotting between periods. The severity of your menstrual cramps can also be affected by lower levels of progesterone, as this hormone can act as a natural pain reliever. So, if levels are low, your cramps are going to be worse (especially when combined with high oestrogen).

One of the main causes of low progesterone, which is also a cause of high estrogen, is high cortisol due to elevated stress levels. Other causes can include the use of birth control pills, and xenoestrogens (which we look at in the next section).

When you look at the link between stress and your hormones, you can see how the hormones can either work together or against each other. If one is out of balance, chances are others are too. For example, DHEA is a steroid hormone that works together with cortisol (our stress hormone) to keep each other in balance. DHEA plays a vital role in producing our sex hormones including progesterone and estrogen, but when cortisol is high DHEA becomes low, impacting on the production of progesterone in the body.

Progesterone can also be stolen by cortisol, a term known as 'pregnenolone steal'. This occurs when the adrenals are so overworked from chronic stress that it breaks down progesterone in order to create more cortisol so the body can deal with the stress. This in turn means that there is more estrogen in the body than progesterone causing estrogen dominance. I'll be looking at stress management in more detail in part 3 when we look at the impact of cortisol on our blood sugar, to avoid repetition.

Another way low progesterone and high estrogen can mess with your menstrual cycle is that it suppresses the production of follicle stimulating hormone (FSH) and causes luteinising hormone (LH) to become more dominant. This can cause ovulation to become irregular or even stop altogether, which then contributes to lower progesterone.

So really, when it comes to our PMS and estrogen dominance, we need to balance our progesterone and estrogen which means we need to find ways to increase our progesterone. So here are some tips on how to raise those progesterone levels:

- **Boost your levels of vitamin B6:** Vitamins B6 helps the body maintain optimal levels of progesterone and helps the liver to break down excess estrogen so it can be removed from the body. I cover vitamin B6 in more detail in part 4, so I'll not focus too much on it here.

- **Take a vitamin C supplement or increase your consumption of vitamin C rich foods such as kiwi, papaya, red bell peppers and cauliflower:** Not only is vitamin C great for the immune system and is a natural antioxidant for the body, it can help make anti stress hormones and can increase progesterone levels. However, best not to go too crazy as too much vitamin C can actually cause elevated estrogen levels in some people.

- **Find ways to lower your stress levels:** Practices such as mindfulness, yoga, meditation, journaling or just getting out and about in nature can help lower those stress levels. The impact of stress and stress management will be covered in more detail in part 3.

- **Maintain a healthy weight:** If you are overweight then you are more prone to estrogen dominance. I'll be explaining why later in this part of the book but high estrogen does cause lower progesterone so weight loss really does help (take it from someone who knows the weight struggles!). However, what you are likely to find is that as you follow the tips in this book and start making those dietary and lifestyle changes, you'll notice the weight loss happening naturally which will be an added bonus if weight is an issue for you.

Beware the Estrogen Imitators

Something we often fail to think about are the toxins that we use and surround ourselves with on a daily basis and it's something I educate clients on in my **28 Day Hormone Reboot Detox** program (you can find this on my website)

We have so many toxins in our environment these days, with over 80,000 different chemicals released into the environment. Toxins are also found in our household and beauty products, in our food supply and even in how we cook and store our food.

When it comes to your hormones and your PMS, some of these toxins will actually imitate estrogen in the body, disrupting your hormone balance and contributing to the severity of your PMS symptoms. These particular types of toxins are known as xenoestrogens.

Xenoestrogens are generally man-made chemicals that are found in many of our everyday products such as household cleaning products, make up, and body care products such as moistures and shower gels but can also be found naturally in certain foods such as soy and beans.

Sources of xenoestrogens include:

- BPA and other types of plastics
- Birth control pills

- Dioxins
- Pesticides
- Food dyes and flavouring agents
- Parabens
- Bleaching agents
- Sunscreens such as those containing benzophenone
- Soy, flax seeds and other beans

The issue with xenoestrogens is that they mimic estrogen in the body, interfering with normal hormone function and therefore increase levels of estrogen. They will either block or over-stimulate the estrogen responders in the body, tricking it into thinking it has more estrogen than it does so the body does not create its own and instead relies on the 'fake' oestrogen or by causing the body to overproduce oestrogen (not great if you're already oestrogen dominant!).

Let's take a look at a few different types of xenoestrogens:

Triclosan
Triclosan is also an estrogen mimicking chemical. It is an anti-bacterial ingredient found in many soaps, lotions, hand creams and in toothpaste. Studies have repeatedly found that this toxin has an impact on our endocrine system which means its bad news for our hormones. It's also been linked to miscarriage, food allergies, and thyroid issues due to increasing T3 levels.

Flame Retardants

Flame retardants often found in upholstered furniture such as sofas and chairs, although no longer allowed in Europe, may still be present in older furnishings. Another estrogen mimicker, exposure to flame retardants will gradually build up those estrogen fakers over time.

BPA and Other Plastics

BPA (Bisphenol-A), found in softened plastics such as water bottles, plastic food containers and canned foods, also contain these estrogen mimicking compounds. Besides being disruptive to your hormones, when you eat/drink food containing it, it can cause your appetite to increase. For those of you looking to lose weight the impact this has is that your increased appetite means you are more likely to snack and overeat, which can lead to further weight gain and even obesity. Bad news for your hormones and your PMS!

Beauty Products

Our skin is our largest organ in the body and one of its roles is to absorb certain products through the hair follicles including creams, fatty substances, essential oils, some medications and a small amount of water. This is why what you put on your skin matters as long-term exposure to chemicals such as parabens, phthalates, artificial fragrances or colours, sodium laurel sulphates or polyethylene glycol will cause major disruption to your hormones and could be a cause of your excess estrogen and the accompanying PMS that comes with it.

Birth Control Pills
Birth control pills contain synthetic hormones which can raise estrogen levels further. This can then contribute to estrogen dominance and put addition strain on the liver which has to try and remove the excess. The scary thing is that most women are put on birth control pills in order to tackle issues like heavy bleeding and PMS, but as you now know … sometimes it can cause more harm than good. It's always worth a chat with your doctor about looking at more natural alternatives.

Our Food Supply
Then there's the hidden estrogen in our food, which are known as phytoestrogens, and include soy, beans, chickpeas and legumes. Soy in all its various forms has been a "should I, shouldn't I" topic for several years and the jury still hasn't come to a clear verdict yet! These phytoestrogens are plant-based estrogens which act as estrogen in the body. There's still a lot of debate out there about the impact of these on oestrogen dominance, as they do tend to also contain phytoestrogens (which can help balance oestrogen levels).

Some people say eating high quantities of these foods worsens oestrogen dominance, whereas a study by Cornell University that looked at breast cancer and the phytoestrogens in soy determined that when eaten in high quantities, phytoestrogens can block estrogen or lower levels found in the blood stream. Personally, I'd say to treat phytoestrogens with caution and eat only in small amounts when estrogen levels are naturally high in the body.

Although it can be difficult to completely avoid all of these things, there are things you can do to help reduce your exposure. Here's some tips to help you reduce your exposure to those estrogen unfriendly toxins:

- **Use a filter jug for your water:** Although most areas have a purification system in place, using a filter jug will help reduce exposure to anything that may still be in your water supply such as lead and bacteria's. In addition to this fluoride and chlorine are often added to water, which although found in such small elements, when consumed on a daily basis may build up over time so a water filter helps reduce your exposure to these.

- **Swap your plastic water bottles and food storage containers for glass ones:** This will help reduce your exposure to plastics such as BPA. You can get sets on Amazon that have glass bottoms and BPA-free plastic lids, I swear by them, plus they are great for meal prepping as the bottoms can go in the oven to reheat or cook food. On the note of reheating food, NEVER microwave food in plastic containers as this will cause the plastic to soften and cause BPA or other toxins to seep into your food.

- **Keep your diet clean and full of fresh produce:** I'm going to be talking about this so much throughout the course of this book that I won't bore you to death with it here but some quick tips are to choose organic foods, especially those on the EWG's dirty dozen list (you'll find the web address in the resources at the end of this book) which are notoriously high in chemicals, or you could even grow your own. Also, go back to traditional cooking with minimal but natural products ... think back to how your grandparents used to cook.

- **Avoid soy and products containing soybean oils or soy additives:** Now, whole soy and fermented soy, such as edamame, miso, tofu and tempeh, are generally okay in moderate amounts however any type of processed soy, such as products containing soybean oil, soy lecithin or modified soy should be avoided.

- **Avoid or limit alcohol, caffeine, and smoking:** This should go without saying, but these all act as toxins in the body and impact on hormone levels as well as putting extra pressure on our liver as the body tries to remove them.

- **Choose natural or 'green' cleaning products:** Be sure to avoid chemical-based products that include chlorine, ammonia, glycol ethers (found in window cleaners), triclosan and fragrances such as phthalates and styrene. Learning to read labels and check for these hidden nasties will serve you and your hormones well in the long run.

- **Look for personal care products that are natural and organic:** Check labels to ensure they are free from parabens, phthalates, toluene (found in many nail polishes), artificial fragrances or colours, sodium laurel sulphates or polyethylene glycol. In fact, why not consider making your own products, there's loads of information out there on the internet for homemade body butters and balms so you'll know exactly what you're putting on your skin.

Why Weight Matters

The biggest complaint I hear from people when they are suffering with any kind of hormone issue, is that they get told 'you need to lose weight'. Have you ever experienced that?

Now, if you're overweight then yes, it will help, but my biggest gripe with this piece of advice given by many professionals is that they don't offer an explanation as to WHY you need to lose weight (plus, it's downright offensive. If we are overweight we already know it, we don't need to be reminded!).

So, let me tell you why your weight matters so you understand the impact it has.

Obesity impacts directly on the sex hormones which means it can raise estrogen levels further. This is bad news if you are already estrogen dominant. It does this by raising levels of insulin in the body which then causes a vicious cycle of overeating, raised blood sugar levels, further weight gain and estrogen dominance. I'll be covering this particular cycle in more depth in part 3.

Another reason as to why weight matters is because our fat cells have the ability to create small amounts of estrogen. Now the issue with a fat cell and weight (or overeating), is that when you overeat the fat cell will swell until it reaches a point it can't swell anymore. It will then divide via a process called mitosis (cell division) meaning the fat cells multiply. If you keep overeating and not burning those consumed calories, you're going to keep creating more fat cells.

In addition to this, is you have a diet and lifestyle that exposes you to a lot of toxins then your fat cells can also be impacted by this. You see, our liver, as awesome as it is, can only remove so much of the toxins (and our excess oestrogen) that it is exposed to. Any excess is sent to our fat cells for 'safe holding' to reduce the risk to our cells. In order to dilute the toxins, the fat cells fill with water which causes them to swell and provide you with that extra padding.

Ultimately, the more fat cells you have, the more estrogen those pesky cells are going to produce which is inevitably going to tip you over into estrogen dominance.

Also, when it comes to your weight, you also need to consider your stress levels because stress triggers cortisol, which again we're going to be looking at in part 3. The point I want to make here is that cortisol can actually cause abdominal fat, which means that stress needs to be addressed if you are looking to lose weight. Not only is abdominal fat the most stubborn fat to get rid of for us women, it's also the type that's going to put you more at risk of other health conditions such as heart disease and stroke.

Now, if you've seen me then you'll know I'm not some stick thin health coach. I do know what it's like to have your weight impact on your hormones and how frustrating it can be to see the scales go up and down each week like a yo-yo despite doing your best to be healthy. It sucks!

You have to remember that weight loss, like addressing this bloody PMS, is a journey. You'll have good days and you'll have bad days but, if you stay true to your goals and do the best you can each day, then you will see results over time. You just need a lot of patience and a good dose of determination.

Also, do NOT fall into the habit of weighing yourself every day. I know so many people who do this and it's so counterproductive. Your body naturally fluctuates by 4lbs every single day plus, if you are exercising as well as making dietary changes, you'll be gaining muscle and toning up. Muscle is denser than fat, so even though the scales may not be showing changes, remember that changes are occurring on the inside.

To get you started in tackling this area, here's my top ten tips to help you with your weight loss:

- **Aim to get 7-8 hours sleep per night:** Many studies have found that getting less than 5 hours sleep significantly increases your weight compared to those who get 8 hours sleep a night, in fact, it was up to 3lbs extra weight for every hour under that 8-hour sleep window! Now I don't know about all of you, but what I'd give to get 8 hours sleep … I'm usually more of a 6-7-hour girl which might explain some of my own personal struggles.

- **Don't fear the healthy fats:** I spent years avoiding fat when I was a member of a well-known sliming group but the fact is, fat doesn't make you fat. It's the processed, high sugar foods we eat that do so make sure you are adding those healthy fats into your diet by eating avocados, using extra virgin olive oil as a salad dressing, or eating nuts and seeds. It's said that healthy fats can actually help promote a healthy weight so, what other excuse do you need!

- **Drink at least 2 litres of water daily:** I know this can seem daunting, and even I struggle with it at times, but staying hydrated with water helps keep hunger cravings at bay, especially if you swap your sugar filled fizzy drinks or pre-packaged fruit juices for water. Hidden sugars in drinks can actually increase your appetite, whereas water (or herbal tea) offers a range of health benefits including helping your liver flush out excess waste, and giving you a clearer complexion.

- **Eat fibre rich foods:** Fibre helps keep you feeling fuller for longer which means you won't want to snack as much. Whole grains including oats and brown rice, chia seeds, beans, legumes and vegetables are all good sources of fibre. Plus, dietary fibre also helps to bind the sex hormones (including estrogen) which helps the body remove the excess as a waste product (okay, I mean it will make you poo out your excess estrogen).

- **Limit your exposure to toxins:** We looked at this in the previous section and I've touched on it in this chapter, but some of those toxins found in our environment and food chain that disrupt our endocrine system can also cause our bodies to not metabolise fat effectively, therefore contributing to weight gain or restricting weight loss.

- **Chew your food properly and eat slowly:** Taking your time to enjoy your food and chew it properly means you will be supporting your digestion. An out of whack digestive tract causing inflammation that's going to further impact on weight loss and estrogen dominance. Plus eating slower means you are less likely to overeat as you are going to be more satisfied with the meal than you would have been if you'd wolfed it down.

- **Don't skip meals, especially breakfast:** When people say breakfast is the most important part of the day they aren't joking. This vital meal actually kick starts your metabolism, helps balance blood sugars and will help keep you feeling full during the morning preventing you from dipping into those biscuits with your mid-morning coffee at work.

- **Avoid sugar, sweets, cakes and pastries:** Seen as I mentioned biscuits, yep those no-good-for-you sugary treats do need to be kicked to the kerb. All refined sugars do are play havoc with blood sugar spikes and drops, which causes you to snack between meals and binge eat as you crave more sugar during the drops. It's hugely disrupting to any weight loss plan.

- **Limit your alcohol intake:** If you can cut it out altogether then great but if not, then try to limit to one alcoholic drink per week. Alcohol is not only a toxin to the body, but it is also a hidden source of sugar which will cause the same issues as sweets, cakes and so on. Think about when you have those boozy nights out and how at the end of it you end up going for a kebab or cheesy chip or the next day you're hungover and binge on carbs and fatty foods … would you have done that if it wasn't for the drink?

- **Add in some exercise:** Yep, the lazy girl who spends most of her time at home on her laptop is telling you to do the exercise. In my defense I walk the dogs twice a day ... and walking IS a form of exercise and I look at my exercise equipment often, so that counts too, right? When it comes to exercise, it doesn't have to be an all-in boot camp style type of exercise, it could be gentle stretching such as yoga (great if you have high stress levels), dancing around in your living room ... whatever you enjoy that gets your body moving. Aim to exercise for 30 minutes at least three times a week because as well as helping tackle your weight by burning some calories, it's a great mood booster too.

Feed Your Flora

There are so many things that can have an impact on your estrogen levels and your PMS as we've been discussing. Your gut flora is the next one that we will be looking at in more detail.

Gut health has only become more spoken about over the last few years, in fact I'd even say it's become a "trendy" topic in the health industry as around 47% of people regularly look for products to help improve their digestive health. It's no surprise than more than 40% of the worldwide population have some form of digestive symptoms, especially when you consider what a 'normal' diet is these days … fatty, processed and genetically modified food and drinks. All of this ends up in the gut!

We have trillions of bacteria, fungi and viruses living in our body, of which over 35,000 types are located in the gut (primarily in the large intestine and colon). Our gut, which also includes the oesophagus, stomach, large and small intestine, plays a critical role in the breakdown and metabolism of food and our absorption of vitamins and nutrients. In addition to this it also plays a role in our mood, immunity and our weight.

Although it can sound a little scary having all these little viruses and bacteria in our body, it is totally normal. However, when the gut becomes dominant in bad bacteria that's when things can go bad. This is known as gut dysbiosis which, in simple terms, is when the microbes (bacteria) in the gut get out of balance. These imbalances can impact on your menstrual cycle, your PMS and your estrogen levels.

When it comes to balancing estrogen levels in the body, particularly via the gut, our estrobolome play a crucial role. The estrobolome are a collection of bacteria in the gut that impacts on whether oestrogen is recirculated or excreted from the body.

If the estrobolome bacteria is healthy and levels are high, excess estrogen is excreted from the body but, if levels of healthy bacteria are low and instead overpopulated with unfriendly bacteria, that bacteria makes an enzyme called beta-glucuronidase which will reactivate the estrogen in your gut. This will then cause that estrogen to be reabsorbed and recirculated in the blood stream.

Bad news if you've already got high levels of estrogen, right?

Gut health can be impacted by the foods we eat, our stress levels, exposure to environmental toxins, the medications we take (did you know that antibiotics for example destroy the good bacteria as well as the bad?), lack of sleep and our alcohol consumption ... all areas we look at throughout the course of this book.

In addition to that, an unhealthy gut can cause further problems such as inflammation in the body that can lead to luteal phase defect, thyroid issues, and other menstrual issues such as PCOS and endometriosis. It's so true when Hippocrates said that all disease begins in the gut!

So how can you start to heal your gut and help improve the population of that good gut flora? Here are eight simple steps to getting started with healing your gut:

- **Reduce your exposure to inflammatory foods:** The most common food groups known to cause inflammation are wheat, dairy, corn, soy and refined sugar. Experiment by paying attention to how you feel after you've eaten any of these then remove one completely from your diet for two weeks, when you reintroduce it (slowly) pay attention to any physical or emotional changes you notice after you've eaten it to see if it's playing havoc with your hormones and/or causing unwanted side effects.

- **Reduce your exposure to inflammatory toxins:** These include alcohol and synthetic drugs including antibiotics, which actually destroy good gut bacteria as well as bad. If you are on or have been on antibiotics be sure to support your gut with some pro-biotics to repopulate the flora.

- **Drink bone broth:** This helps with rebuilding the good gut bacteria and supporting it. Save the bones from your roast dinners and boil them up adding vegetables too if you like for extra flavour, then strain the liquid and each day drink a cup or two of it just like you would a cup of tea (but perhaps without the milk and sugar, I really don't think that would work so well).

- **Add zinc rich foods or a zinc supplement into your diet:** There's more information on zinc in part 4 as this is a great PMS buster too, but when it comes to your gut, zinc also helps repair damaged cells so can be healing for the gut lining.

- **Chew your food properly:** We so often eat in a rush, I know I am often guilty of this, but slowing down to take the time to enjoy your food and chew it thoroughly will improve your gut health in the long run as the digestive system can then break down your food properly. By chewing your food properly your digestive system won't have larger chunks of food passing through it which can be a contributing factor to issues such as leaky gut.

- **Eat fibre-rich foods:** Foods that are full in fibre include whole wheat, chickpeas, beans and lentils, fruits and vegetables. If your diet isn't fibre rich then do increase the amount of fibre you eat slowly and be sure to increase your water consumption at the same time too to prevent constipation.

- **Add in some probiotic-rich and fermented foods:** Foods such as plain, full-fat yogurt, kefir, sauerkraut, kimchi, miso and pickles - these will help repopulate the good bacteria in your gut and help to improve its over health.

- **Eat prebiotic resistant foods:** These include lentils, chickpeas and cooked and cooled potatoes which will stimulate the good bacteria and help maintain the levels of the bad bacteria so they don't get out of control.

Look After Your Liver

The liver is the second largest organ in the body and it is the bodies primary organ of detoxification.

Everything we eat, drink, inhale or absorb through our skin is filtered through the liver so that harmful byproducts can be filtered from the blood and removed as a waste product. It also removes excess estrogen from the body, which is why we are talking about it here.

But jeez, don't we often put our livers under a lot of stress through binge drinking (which we have all done at some point in our life, I'm sure … or is that just me?), over indulging in sugary and fatty foods, the environmental toxins that surround us in everyday life and the plethora of skin creams, lotions and potions that we use on an almost daily basis!

Whenever we exposure ourselves to any of these toxins the liver must work at removing them to help keep our blood clean and keep our bodies functioning as they should. It does this using a two-phase mode of detoxification.

In the first phase, the liver transforms the toxin into a chemical that it can process in the second stage. These toxins at this point are generally fat-soluble in nature so the liver needs to convert these into a water-soluble form that can be processed during stage two of the detoxification process.

As the liver then moves into phase two, these now water-soluble toxins are ready to be excreted from the body through either the urine (as it passes through the kidneys) or our bowel movements (via bile that is released into the intestinal tract).

However, sometimes this process doesn't work as it should causing the toxins to be recirculated into the blood. When that happens, one of the common symptoms of a dysfunctional liver is PMS. In addition to that, if the liver is dysfunctional, and therefore unable to do its job correctly, this can lead to or worsen estrogen dominance.

But what causes the liver to stop working effectively?

The primary, and most common, cause can be that the liver is simply overwhelmed. If you take a lot of prescription medication, drink a lot of alcohol, smoke or take recreational drugs then the liver is generally unable to keep up with the toxic load so circulates these toxins back into the blood until it is able to handle them.

Another cause can be that the liver becomes sluggish due to a buildup of toxins over time, such as environmental toxins or a buildup of free radicals which are produced during phase one liver detoxification and can cause damage our cells.

Other issues that may impact on liver function include inflammation in the GI tract, inflammation in the liver from alcohol, liver toxic medication, metabolic syndrome which is a result of blood sugar imbalance (we look at this in part 3), or gallbladder dysfunction where the gallbladder becomes sluggish or slow to empty.

The gallbladder works alongside the liver, so if you've got estrogen dominance you don't want a sluggish gallbladder as this plays a crucial role in metabolising our sex hormones and keeping excess estrogen and our weight in check. Are you noticing how everything is so closely linked when it comes to estrogen and PMS?

To help improve your liver and gallbladder function you need to decrease your toxic load and support your liver by improving your diet and lifestyle (which is what you've already been starting to do as you work through this book).

To recap on how to reduce your toxic load here's some key pointers so you don't have to flick back to the previous sections:

- ♦ Avoid alcohol, caffeine, smoking and recreational drugs. Not only will this help prevent liver overload, but it is also beneficial for your gut and will prevent gut bacteria from attacking the liver.

- Filter your water to remove hidden chemicals and bacteria.

- Ventilate your home by either using an air purifier or opening your windows as often as possible.

- Avoid plastics such as plastic wrap, plastic lined cans, and swap plastic food containers to glass versions to reduce your exposure to BPA and other plastics that can disrupt your endocrine system.

- Use chemical free beauty products - check the labels to ensure they are free from parabens and other nasty chemicals, and to check they do not contain artificial fragrances.

- Swap chemical-based household cleaning products for natural brands, it's more expensive but your hormones will thank you in the long run.

To support your liver through diet and lifestyle here are some simple tips to help get it back in tip-top condition:

- Take supplements that support liver function such as, B-vitamins, vitamins A, C, D and E, and N-acetyl cysteine which is a pre-cursor for glutathione (the master antioxidant). The

B-Complex is especially important as vitamin B6 helps the liver to break down estrogen.

- Eat liver supportive and antioxidant foods such as sweet potato, carrots, beets, citrus, melon, strawberries, avocados and cruciferous vegetables such as broccoli and cabbage.

- Eat high-quality proteins such as eggs, fish, organ meats (if you're brave enough, I'm not!) and bone broth as these contain amino-acids that will support phase two of liver detoxification.

- Support your GI tract with fibre rich foods and work on improving your gut health as we discussed in the previous section '*Feed your Flora*'.

- Manage your stress levels. This is covered in more detail in Part 3 but this will help decrease the over-production of cortisol which will also help support liver function.

- Use herbs that support your liver such as chlorophyll and turmeric. I personally tend to have a chlorophyll drink on an evening before bed, simply add 1 teaspoon of good quality liquid chlorophyll and the juice of half a lemon to a glass of water, stir and drink. The first time you have it, it may taste weird (I thought it was like drinking pond water ... not that I've ever drunk pond water!) but you soon get used to it and in fact, now, I quite enjoy it.

- Support the remove of waste by breaking a sweat. It's a perfect excuse to indulge in a sauna or steam room on a regular basis, or depending on what phase of your menstrual cycle you are at do it through some intense exercise.

Alternatively, you may want to help support your liver and give yourself a clean slate on which to build your PMS healing efforts by doing my ***28 Day Hormone Reboot Detox*** first, as this will help to remove toxic build up and eliminate toxins being held in the fat cells.

P.S. It isn't some crazy juice cleanse, it's an educational detox program that involves real, solid foods! If you've not learnt anything about me yet, let me assure you I am NOT a juice only girl, so I'd never push something on you that I'm not willing or haven't done myself.

Part 3: Glucose Intolerance

What is Glucose Intolerance?

Glucose intolerance and insulin resistance are very closely linked. You'll notice that when I'm looking at addressing this, I mention insulin resistance quite a lot as tackling this will help to tackle glucose intolerance.

To explain the difference, insulin resistance is when the cells in the muscle, fat tissue and liver are less able to remove glucose from your blood, this causes blood glucose levels to rise and results in glucose intolerance which can lead to metabolic syndrome. This is why you have to tackle insulin resistance first, so you can prevent it developing into glucose intolerance.

Although the digestive system and gut health play a role in glucose management, which is why it's so important to look after that gut flora, the pancreas plays a critical role in the process of keeping blood glucose levels stable. Let me explain how it all works …

When we eat food, the pancreas releases insulin so it can prepare the cells to absorb the sugar. When the levels of sugar go down, the pancreas then releases glucagon which tells the cells to stop taking in the sugar. This helps to ensure that blood sugar levels don't go too low. Insulin resistance occurs when the messages to absorb the sugar are sent but ignored by the cells, and so the sugars stay in the blood stream.

We have several cells in the body that respond to insulin; muscles, liver and fat tissue. These are the major players in energy storage and usage so are generally impacted the most when insulin resistance kicks in but, the brain can be impacted too as some of the cells in there are actually dependent on blood sugars. When the brain becomes impacted by insulin resistance it has an impact on not only the reproductive system but also our food intake, weight and memory function.

Early signs of insulin resistance include that sluggish morning feeling where there just isn't enough coffee available to get you up and going, midafternoon sugar cravings and the need for a sweet treat that MUST be satisfied after dinner in the evening.

I actually blame the foundations of these evening craving on our childhoods ... do you ever remember being told you couldn't have that pudding if you didn't eat all your dinner? So, you would force down your dinner just so you could have that pudding ... early signs of classical conditional taking place and the roots of our eating habits, which as I'm sure you know, can be bloody hard to break (especially when combined with hormonal imbalances).

Other symptoms of insulin resistance include fatigue, brain fog, abdominal fat, sugar cravings and feeling tired after meals, but often people don't realise they have it in the early stages. It's generally only noticed when it develops into a more serious condition which is why it is so important to be mindful when it comes to your sugar consumption.

But insulin resistance isn't the end point. It's only the starting point of blood sugar issues and can lead on to Type 2 Diabetes and even metabolic syndrome, one of the leading causes of death, which has been linked to strokes, heart disease, PCOS and certain types of cancer.

But how does your blood sugar relate to your PMS?

Our ovaries have insulin receptors and excess insulin will cause them to make androgens (male hormones) instead of pro-fertility hormones which is why it causes so many issues for our reproductive system. Too much testosterone (one of the 'male' hormones) can disrupt or stop ovulation completely throwing your cycle well and truly off balance. It also ramps up cortisol production (our stress hormone) which can increase visceral fat.

In addition to this, our PMS is directly affected by insulin resistance as it contributes to estrogen dominance. Although estrogen is primarily produced in the ovaries, insulin resistance can cause the peripheral muscle which converts testosterone into estrogen to overproduce estrogen. This occurs because excess insulin causes the muscles to grow which in turn means it converts even more testosterone to estrogen. Yay, hormones ... NOT!

But worry not ... insulin resistance does not have to develop into something more sinister. Just like all the other things we've looked at so far, it can be addressed and managed. Remember, YOU hold the power to heal your body.

Let's take a look at some of the main causes of insulin resistance:

- **Obesity:** Fat in the body plays a huge role in our metabolism and our blood sugar balance. When the fat stores sugar (or excess food) but doesn't use it, that puts stress on our body. It can cause the body to release inflammatory proteins which increases insulin resistance. We've talked about weight when we looked at estrogen dominance so if you need to refresh, head back to '*Why Weight Matters*' in part 2.

- **Diet:** As we've covered many times in this book, what you eat really does impact on your hormones and your PMS. I'll be covering this is more detail too, especially the specific points when it comes to blood sugar balancing.

- **Inflammation:** Sugar causes inflammation, that's a fact, and inflammation that affects our insulin resistance (and therefore our PMS) can occur in either the gut or our fatty tissue. I'll be sharing more about this with you in this section of the book.

- **Stress:** I've mentioned stress so many times as it plays a major role in almost every aspect of hormone imbalance and your PMS. We are going to be discussing how this can impact on your blood sugar levels and look at ways to manage those stress levels so you can get back in control of those PMS mood swings and, support your blood sugar balance.

- **Lack of Sleep:** Can you really sleep yourself healthy? Erm, yes, you can, although many of us don't actually get enough sleep. In this section I'll be looking at how sleep affects your insulin resistance and ways to promote a good night's sleep.

- **Toxins:** There are so many toxins around us in our everyday life and many of these can impact on insulin sensitivity levels. We looked at reducing our toxic exposure back in Part 2, as many of the recommendations are the same I won't repeat it all here. If you need to refresh your knowledge on toxins revisit *Watch out for Fake Estrogens* in part 2.

- **The Wrong Type of Exercise:** Oh my god, I'm saying it … exercise may NOT be good for you! Now, I've always been a firm believer you shouldn't run unless you're being chased (guess I'm a gonner if the zombie apocalypse ever happens) but it can be true. Exercise has the power to either improve or worsen your insulin resistance. I'll be telling you more about this later in this part of the book.

So now you know what needs to be addressed when it comes to blood sugar balance and your PMS, so are you ready to get started?

Let's Talk Sugar

Before we dive on in to balancing blood sugar through diet, lets pause a moment to discuss sugar and all its hidden forms, because trust me when I tell you … it's in almost everything and it's hugely addictive.

In fact, sugar consumption triggers the release of various chemicals in the brain and when you take away the sugar, you can actually suffer withdrawal symptoms similar to that of someone giving up drugs or alcohol! Scary, right?

Sugar tends to be classified as a carbohydrate, but not all carbohydrates are equal as you are about to discover. Sugar is a major disruptor to your hormones and your blood sugar levels, it causes inflammation in the body, it makes us gain weight and of course, the reason you're reading this book, is that it plays a role in the development of your PMS symptoms.

Sugar is the simplest form of carbohydrate and includes the three main players: glucose, fructose, and lactose as well as many other forms of sugar. In fact, there are so many different names that sugar is disguised as, and if you start checking labels, you'll notice the one key thing about most of these, it's that they end in -ose.

Sugar consumption causes an immediate spike in blood sugars whereas complex carbohydrates, such as starches and fibre, slowly release the energy over time. This rapid spike caused by sugar (which has little nutritional value, in the case of refined sugars) actually promotes fat storage and causes high blood sugar levels. If these levels are not controlled, it can actually put your body into an anabolic state which will actually stop your body burning fat for energy - bad news if weight loss is on your list of areas to address.

In addition to that, when you get the blood sugar drop that follows a blood sugar spike, you seek out foods that will quickly restore those elevated blood sugar levels. Yep, it's another vicious cycle; eat sugar, blood sugar rises, blood sugar drops, you crave sugar.

It's not all doom and gloom though, we do need some sugars in our diet for energy. Our bodies are designed to deal with small amounts of sugar however, in today's modern world, we are surrounded by the stuff. From pre-packaged fruit juices that are designed to appeal to the health conscious, to the processed foods that are developed to 'make our lives easier' such as jarred sauces, salad dressings, ketchup and certain canned foods, to the fast food that's consumed far more often than it should be, and even in that chocolate that we crave when we have PMS.

The problem that we are all having, is that is we are eating far more of it than we should be. In fact, it's been said that the average adult consumes around 22 teaspoons of sugar a day and the average child consumes 32 teaspoons a day. If those figures are correct, what that means is we are actually setting our children up to have the same problems in the future that we have now.

So, let's look at the different types of carbohydrate-based sugars found in our food that we need to be mindful of:

- **Monosaccharides:** These are simple, single chain sugars including fructose, which is found in fruit, soft drinks, sweeteners and syrup, and glucose, which is found in fruit, sweeteners, grains and potatoes. It's the most natural form of sugar.

- **Disaccharides:** These are sugars that are made up of two sugar chains and include sucrose, found in dried fruits and refined sugar, lactose, found in milk and dairy produce, and maltose, which is found in molasses.

- **Polysaccharides:** These are long chains of connecting monosaccharides (so lots of single sugars all connected) and are commonly known as complex carbohydrates.

Whole grains, starchy vegetables and legumes are all polysaccharides.

Monosaccharides can be used for energy almost immediately by absorbing it into the blood stream, whereas disaccharides and polysaccharides need to be broken down into monosaccharides which is why polysaccharides offer slow releasing energy. Energy that isn't needed is stored in the bodies short term energy supplies to be used later, but when we eat more sugar than the stores can hold, the rest will get stored away in our long-term stores which are located in … our fat cells! In other words, unused sugar becomes fat … oh, yay!

Consumption of monosaccharides and disaccharides should be limited as they are known to contribute to blood sugar imbalance and inflammation in the body. Fructose is also often classed as toxic by the liver and, as we looked at in the last part of the book, we may need our liver to focus on ridding the body of excess estrogen so we don't want to overload or distract it from that job.

Now you've got a little background on the role of sugar when it comes to your PMS, let's move on to ways we can address it and regain control of any blood sugar imbalances you may have. Oh, and even if you think you don't have blood sugar issues, remember that you may have insulin resistance without knowing it, but either way prevention is better than cure so, the advice in this part of the book is still just as valid for you as anyone else.

Balance Blood Sugars Through Diet

As we discussed when we just looked at sugar, diet is one of the quickest and easiest ways to regain control over blood sugar imbalance and I'm going to discuss each of the three major food groups with you (carbohydrates, proteins and fats) so you have a better knowledge of how they all work when it comes to your blood sugars.

Carbohydrates

When it comes to carbohydrates, it's the processed and refined carbohydrates that are the biggest culprits for causing disruption to your blood sugar levels and your hormone issues. They increase inflammation in the body, make insulin resistance worse, and increase the production of cortisol and estrogen in the body ... and haven't we already been discussing minimising many of these already as part of your journey towards regaining control over your PMS?

These processed and refined carbohydrates are by far the poorest quality and should be heavily reduced or cut out altogether because, as we looked at when we discussed sugars, they get processed immediately causing those blood sugar spikes and if that excess energy is not used, it stores as glycogen in the liver or, as fat in our tissues, both of which can also impact on estrogen dominance.

Foods to be especially mindful of include white sugar, white flour, corn products, white pasta/rice/bread, and baked goods such as cakes and pastries. Chances are, it's all your favourite foods, as that sugar is an addictive little bugger!

Instead, opt for low GI fruits and vegetables, resistant starches, which are fruits and vegetables that resist digestion (this means they don't break down in the stomach or intestines so, are a great source of fibre) including sweet potatoes, squash, legumes, green bananas, beans and peas and grains such as oats, wheat, barley and rye (as long as you aren't sensitive to gluten). If you are sensitive to gluten, or even if you're not, then quinoa, brown rice, millet and buckwheat make a great alternative.

Proteins

Protein is an essential structural component in hormone production so we need to have enough of it in our diet, yet many of us don't. It also contains barely any sugar which means it isn't going to have any negative impact on your blood sugar levels.

In fact, it's been said that one protein-only meal per day can be hugely beneficial for people suffering with insulin resistance as it will prevent the blood sugars from spiking and falling as much. What better excuse is there for bacon, sausage and eggs for breakfast!

Although it's said a low protein diet, of under 50g protein a day, can help decrease insulin levels, it can also stimulate your stress response and increase body fat which will have a negative impact on blood sugar management and other areas that impact on your PMS. Due to this, I'd say be careful of any overly-restrictive and 'fad' diets, instead look at your own personal needs and requirements. There are many apps and online calculators that you can use to help calculate your macronutrient requirements.

Animal produce, especially organ meats, if you can stomach them, are generally the best choice for protein as these contain all the 8 amino acids that our bodies cannot create on their own. Other good sources that are also suitable for vegan or vegetarians include spirulina, lentils, quinoa, buckwheat. Brown rice, beans and peas are also proteins but work best when teamed with another protein as they are not classed as 'complete' on their own.

Fats

I've touched upon healthy fats a few times already, I'm sure, but our hormones are produced from fat and cholesterol so we don't want to miss out on this vital nutrient. Despite years of the media and their marketing campaigns ramming fat-free and low-fat products down our necks and claiming they are 'healthier' for us. Even I got duped by that one for years when I was a member (and later a consultant) for a slimming group that heavily promoted fat-free products.

Fats helps to balance our hormones, improve our menstrual cycles, can improve our weight struggles, support our brain function and decrease inflammation in our bodies. So, why are we so fearful of it when all we have to do is swap those bad fats for good fats?

Let me explain a little bit about the different types of fat:

Saturated fats are fats that are generally solid at room temperature such as butter, lard and coconut oil. **Unsaturated fats** can be monounsaturated such as avocado and olive oil, or polyunsaturated such as salmon, flax seeds and walnuts.

Then, there's our **omega fatty acids** that are essential for normal function, yet unable to be produced by our bodies, so if we aren't getting them in our diet, we risk deficiency (we look at these more in part 4). You need to make sure you are adding these into your diet.

The fats you need to be avoiding and heavily reducing your consumption of include **rancid fats**, which are commonly found in processed oils such as canola oil, sunflower oil, and soy, and **trans fats**, found in baked goods and fried foods. These fats are known endocrine disruptors which interfere with our sex hormones and increase inflammation in the body.

Here are some tips to help get you started on the right track towards getting those blood sugars back in balance through your diet:

- **Check the Sugar Content on Labels:** This was something I encouraged my ladies to do during a sugar detox challenge as it's a real eye opener when you start looking at labels. A huge shocker for me was the Maggi cook-in bags for chicken that I used to use quite often … it contained about 33g of sugar per 100g which means it was one third sugar! Needless to say, they are no longer a household staple as I can season meat with herbs and spices instead of sugar.

- **Eat a Low GI Diet:** This will help keep your blood sugars more stable and help keep you fuller for longer. When it comes to the GI numbers, lower is better, it's like a percentage. If a food product has a GI of 95 that means it's going to raise your blood sugars by 95% whereas a food that has a GI rating of 12 will only raise blood sugars by 12%. A quick Google search and you'll easily find several guides giving you the GI ratings of many foods.

- **Have a High Fat, High Protein Breakfast:** This will help stabilise morning blood sugars. Foods such as sausage, eggs, avocado or greens make a great choice. How about a sausage and spinach omelette? Or perhaps avocado and egg on whole meal toast, or even bacon, sausage, eggs, tomato and mushrooms … yummy!

- **Always Eat Carbohydrates with Protein and Fats:** This includes snacks! This helps prevent blood sugar spikes. Plus, proteins and fats are broken down much slower by the body so help to slow down and draw out insulin levels, which means more stable blood sugars.

- **Choose your Carbs Wisely:** Swap out simple and refined carbs for complex carbs as these will release the glucose slowly, preventing you from getting those blood sugar spikes and drops that have you reaching for the snack cupboard. Focus on wholegrain, fibre-rich and starchy carbohydrates such as brown rice, quinoa, sweet potatoes and oats.

- **Increase your Consumption of Healthy Fats as you Lower Carbohydrates:** Eating less carbohydrates can help to stabilise blood sugar levels, so as well as choosing your carbs with care be sure to increase your healthy fats in order to help keep you feeling fuller for longer. In addition to this, less carbs will also help shift abdominal fat which will lower your risk of other health related conditions such as metabolic syndrome but please, don't go for a carbohydrate restrictive 'fad' diet as you do need those carbs for energy. It's all about balance and moderation.

- **Consider a Mediterranean Diet:** They say the Mediterranean diet is one of the healthiest with its abundance of healthy fats, quality protein, wild caught fish and seasonal vegetables. Think back to the last holiday you had and the foods you may have eaten there; Greek salads, fish with boiled potatoes and salad in a lemon juice and olive oil dressing, hearty stews packed with root vegetables, grilled chicken kebabs. I don't know about you, but I'm getting hungry and craving a holiday thinking about it! The Mediterranean diet is also often acknowledged as being one of the best for blood sugar balancing.

- **Spice Up Your Life:** I bet you so wanted to sing that like the Spice Girls did! Certain spices can help with blood sugar management so, I challenge you to get creative with your seasonings and your use of them. Two spices that are must haves for blood sugar balancing are curcumin and cinnamon. Curcumin is the active ingredient in turmeric and is an anti-inflammatory often used in Indian cooking which has an indirect effect on insulin through decreasing inflammation in the muscles, and Cinnamon makes insulin receptors more responsive, helping to absorb energy into the muscles as well as decreasing inflammation in the fat cells.

- **Take Supplements that Support Blood Sugar Management:** Although I look at this in more detail in the next part, certain supplements can help with blood sugar management, especially if you are struggling with dietary changes (but diet is always the best way to do this). Magnesium, Vitamin D, Chromium, and Inulin can all help with improving your insulin sensitivity.

- **Drink Plenty of Water:** Often we mistake dehydration for hunger. Drinking plenty of water can help keep those sugar cravings at bay which will help manage blood sugar levels in the long run.

Reduce Inflammation

As I mentioned earlier, inflammation in the body has been found to contribute to insulin resistance and the development of glucose intolerance, as well as having been linked to PMS symptoms such as mood swings, abdominal cramps, bloating, cravings and breast pain.

One study by Gold, Wells and Razor (2016) determined that the inflammation causing your PMS is down to elevated hs-CRP levels (High-Sensitivity C-reactive protein), a biomarker for inflammation. Although that's a bit high-science for me and this book, in simple terms, studies have shown inflammation to have an impact on PMS.

That same study also determined that women who were overweight or obese were more likely to experience these elevated levels so again, weight management has a crucial role to play in addressing inflammation, blood sugar balance, and PMS.

In order to understand why weight matters, you need to understand the ways in which inflammation can occur in the body. Inflammation occurs in two different ways; in the adipose tissues which would explain why women with weight issues are more likely to experience PMS symptoms, and inflammation in the gut microbiome.

Chronic Inflammation in the Adipose (Fat) Tissues

This is directly linked to obesity, especially in people who have increased abdominal fat, and as we spoke about before when we looked at why weight matters, that excess fat is also going to increase your estrogen. Isn't it crazy how everything interlinks so much … if one system is out of order the others follow too!

Part of our immune system includes immune cells known as macrophages, these macrophages can be anti-inflammatory or pro-inflammatory. When it comes to chronic inflammation in the adipose tissue, the number of pro-inflammatory macrophages have been shown to increase in white adipose tissue in people who are obese (Shimobayashi, et al. 2018). This, then promotes tissue inflammation that can lead to glucose intolerance.

In case that's made your head boggle, in simple terms, this means the fat cells release pro-inflammatory molecules that will prevent insulin from clearing the sugar from the blood and putting it in the cells that require it, therefore blocking insulin from doing its job properly and causing inflammation in the body.

Chronic Inflammation in the Gut Microbiome

We've spoken about our gut bacteria in the last part of the book, but looking after your gut health is more than just about balancing estrogen.

When the gut bacteria are properly balanced it helps to maintain blood sugar levels, our weight, and promotes a 'normal' appetite but, when it's not balanced it allows the overgrowth of inflammatory bacteria which can lead to leaky gut. The combination of leaky gut and that bad bacteria causes obesity, fatty liver and insulin resistance. It can also cause our fatty tissues to be broken down, which despite sounding like a good thing will actually cause further inflammation in the body.

In addition to this, a study by Roomruangwong, et al. (2019) found that our antibody levels and pathogen markers in our gut bacteria vary drastically throughout our menstrual cycle, peaking towards the end of our luteal phase. They summarised that the increased load of gram-negative bacteria in the gut that occurs at the end of the cycle (in the luteal phase) is associated to premenstrual symptoms including fatigue, anxiety, breast swelling and food cravings. Even more reason to look after your gut!

I feel like I'm starting to sound like a broken record as I have mentioned vicious cycles so many times already in this book but, when it comes to blood sugar management we see that vicious cycle raise its head again. When you have unbalanced blood sugars you have increased sugar cravings, this promotes bacterial imbalances in the gut which causes further inflammation and causes weight gain, and weight gain causes more sugar cravings.

So hopefully, you can see how important it is to get your blood sugar balanced in order to improve all other aspects of your health, especially your PMS, and break that cycle once and for all.

The tips we covered in Part 2 on *Why Weight Matters* and *Feed Your Flora* will give you advice on ways to tackle these particular areas of concern. In addition to that, everything I'm covering in this book will also help you work towards balancing inflammation in the body.

Stress Less

You've seen me mention stress management a few times throughout this book and that's because it plays such a huge role in our hormone health, in our PMS, and, because it also has a direct impact on insulin regulation, which is why I have saved it until now to discuss.

We live in a high stress world where we work long hours, manage our homes, our families, try to have a social life ... let's face it, as women we try to do everything but we simply can't keep up to all the demands and expectations placed upon us (despite thinking we can). This just causes stress to build up in our bodies whether we realise it or not. We are only human after all and we often forget that.

As women, we stress about everything and anything, from the little things like being stuck in a traffic jam, or when its PMS week and we stress for absolutely no reason at all, or just because our partner gave us a funny look (and needs to dodge flying pans). We stress about money, our jobs, what we heard on the news, that we don't have enough time, all the little 'jobs' we didn't manage to get done that day ... are you getting my point here?

In fact, around 80% of doctor's appointments are stress-related and, statistics by the American Institute of Stress showed that stress affects sleep in

48% of people, mental health in a whopping 73% of people and physical health in 77% of people.

However, stress can come from a variety of sources. It can be physical stress such as an injury, exposure to extreme temperatures, malnutrition or illness, or it can be a psychological stress such as fear, conflict, anger, grief or worry. Our bodies are designed to cope with short term stress, this goes back to caveman days where man would see a monster and need to run to save his life but today, we live in a state of ongoing and constant stress.

But, all we do when we live in this state of high stress is cause a constant release of cortisol into our blood stream which has a detrimental effect on our hormones and our blood sugar management. It also puts a massive strain on our adrenal glands and can lead to adrenal fatigue, a far more serious consequence of chronic stress.

When we look at how cortisol and insulin work together they actually ramp each other up like two naughty children egging each other on. Too much insulin causes the body to produce more cortisol (our main stress hormone) which contributes to insulin resistance. Insulin resistance means the pancreas tries to create more insulin, which increases cortisol and so yet another vicious cycle begins. Yep, there's me and those vicious cycles again ... you'll be dreaming about them I'm sure!

The more cortisol we have, the more abdominal fat we also accumulate, which feeds into that chronic inflammation we just spoke about. This then causes the fatty tissues to create more inflammatory proteins, makes the cells less sensitive to insulin, AND increases our appetite.

In addition to this, stress has a huge impact on our menstrual cycle. We need a certain balance of DHEA and cortisol so when cortisol is high, DHEA goes down causing our body to produce less estrogen and progesterone. I also mentioned to you, back in part 2, how cortisol can steal progesterone from the body to cope in times of stress or block it leading to estrogen dominance. So, you see, its crucial to manage your stress levels in order to manage your hormone levels and your PMS symptoms.

Here's my top tips for tackling those stressful situations in your life (sadly, I can't help remove the kids or the partner!):

- ♦ **Self-Care is Key:** You NEED to take time out for rest and relaxation, this should be a non-negotiable. Great stress busting self-care practices include meditation, yoga, gratitude, journaling, indulging in a bubble bath, or spending time in nature. Whatever gives you that feeling of peace and harmony is what you need to prioritise into your life.

- **Don't Be Afraid to Delegate or Ask for Help:** It's okay to ask for help. You're not superwoman ... and even if you are, everyone needs a little help sometimes. At home, don't be afraid to delegate tasks, set the kids chores or create a schedule. At work, delegate tasks or if you are self-employed, look at ways you can outsource certain tasks, whether that's hiring a virtual assistant or employing a cleaner once a week (I highly recommend the latter if the thought of cleaning makes you want to have a meltdown, as I know it does for me!).

- **Get Adequate Sleep:** Several studies have found that if you don't get enough sleep, your body produces more cortisol. It does this to give you that boost of energy to help get you up and going in the morning. I'll be coving some tips on how to get better sleep in the next section.

- **Change Your Mindset:** All too often stress can be perceived as worse than it is. Learning to identify where the thought came from and giving it a new story can be key. For example, if you are looking at a stressful situation in a negative way, instead try looking at it as a challenge or lesson to be learnt. Try to find the positive in every situation as this will help to make minor stresses easier to deal with. And, if you can't change it, why stress about it?

- **Spend Time with People who make you Feel Good:** As humans we are designed for social connection. It's one of the things I struggled with the most when I moved to Portugal and still do from time to time (even as an introvert). But, as humans we are designed to want social interaction (unless it's our PMS week) so spending time with people who make you feel good can actually decrease stress levels. Equally you need to avoid those people who don't make you feel good or drain your energy ... we call those the energy vampires, you know the people who literally suck the life out of you when you are around them. Failing that, get a cat or dog as its been proven that stroking them releases our happy hormones and reduces stress levels too.

- **Take a Break from Social Media & the News:** A huge cause of stress, or dissatisfaction with our own lives, comes courtesy of our social media platforms. We spend so much time scrolling through our feeds, looking at all the influencers and people with their fantastic lifestyles and glamorous looks, and it makes us feel like sh*t about ourselves and our own lives. In addition to this, if you wake up every morning and watch or read the news, STOP! All you are doing is starting your day on a negative as the news is ALWAYS doom and gloom. I challenge you to take a 24-hour break from social media and/or the news and take note of any differences in how you feel mentally afterwards, I think you'll be surprised.

Sleep Yourself Healthy

Did you realise that when we sleep our bodies are repairing all the damage of the day? Yet many of us fail to get adequate sleep, which has been shown to be a vital component when it comes to both blood sugar management, our weight and, in turn, our PMS.

In fact, we are so often trying to squeeze as much into our days as possible that we end up burning the candle at both ends and ultimately, burning ourselves out. Have a think about what time you get up and what time you go to bed ... then once in bed, do you fall straight asleep? Does your mind struggle to switch off and keep you awake with whirring thoughts? Or, do you wake often through the night?

There have been many studies over the years that look at sleep and its impact on our hormones. One study found that just four days of sleeping less than 5 hours per night increased insulin resistance in HEALTHY people by 30% ... so imagine what it's like if you're not healthy!

In addition to the impact on insulin resistance, lack of sleep has also been linked to heart disease, obesity and fertility issues. Not getting enough shut eye will increase your appetite and contribute to inflammation in the body (which you are probably also working on now so even more reason to get that early night you've been promising yourself).

In fact, when it comes to weight, multiple studies have found that the average weight difference between people who got 8 hours sleep and those who got less was 3lbs for every hour under the 8-hour benchmark. Hand me the sleeping pills ... I'll see you in a week when I've got a figure like Jennifer Aniston!

On a serious note however, our bodies run on a circadian rhythm that stems all the way back to caveman days. We had a biological rhythm of sleeping when it was dark and waking when it was daylight. Light is the main component involved in this process, but thanks to the amount of technology and artificial lights we are now surrounded by, light signals have distorted our circadian rhythm and overstimulated our brains.

When it comes to insulin resistance and your PMS, it's worth noting that ALL hormones in the body are affected by insulin which is why you might notice that your sleep is impacted when its PMS time. A study by Jehan, et al (2016) found that women with PMDD (the severest form of PMS) had a decreased response to and lower levels of secretion of melatonin, our wind down and sleep hormone. They also determined that sleep disturbances were also caused by increased levels of progesterone during the luteal phase.

With this in mind, and the fact that your PMS may really screw with your sleep and worsen insulin resistance, its vitally important to get a sleep routine in place to help you unwind before bed and help to promote a good night's rest. So here are my top tips for supporting your sleep:

- **Stick to a regular bedtime**: Your body responds better to a routine, so even if you feel like you can't sleep, still head to bed at that pre-determined time. Even just lying there resting can help your body to wind down, or listen to some soothing music or a guided meditation. I listen to a chakra guided meditation sometimes and it always helps me fall asleep, as focusing on picturing the meditation distracts my mind from all the racing thoughts.

- **Create a bedtime ritual:** You probably have a morning one without realising, I know I do. I get up, go to the toilet, brush my teeth and go for coffee … in that exact order, every morning. So, getting yourself wound down for bed using a process like you do when you gear up on a morning is just as important. Some things you could try include in a bedtime routine are:

    - Meditating

- ☐ Journaling (keep it positive and include what you are grateful for that day)
- ☐ Gentle stretching or Yoga
- ☐ Diffusing some essential oils
- ☐ Relaxing in an Epsom salts bath then getting snuggly in your pjs
- ☐ Reading in bed with a cup of herbal tea, such as chamomile

♦ **Make your bedroom an inviting space:** Clear out the clutter. Make sure your bed is made, the pillows are plush, sheets are luxurious. Perhaps you want scented candles (keep them away from the curtains though!) to create a beautiful aroma, some potted plants to help oxygenate the room and some gentle, soft lighting for ambience. This room wants to be the place you really want to retreat to. Oh, and ban the electronics, especially the TV which men seem obsessed with getting in there. The best saying I ever heard was: "The bedroom should be for sleeping and sex." Make it your boudoir, make it as extravagant or exotic as you like, or keep it simple, clean and crisp. Whatever works for you.

♦ **Have an electronics curfew:** Artificial lights and the lights emitted by television, mobile phones and computers are high on the blue light spectrum. This not only overstimulate our brain but just one night of blue light exposure can cause you to have slower metabolism and decreased energy the next day. Stop using electronic devices around 1-2 hours before bed and put them on silent so they don't disturb you when you are trying to rest. There is nothing worse than the ping of a message at stupid o'clock in the middle of the night.

- **Stop eating 2 hours before bed:** Eating just before bed actually activates your digestive system which disturbs your sleep. In addition to this, it can cause blood sugar spikes followed by a blood sugar crash that can also disturb your sleep.

- **Avoid alcohol and caffeine:** I used to believe that the wine helped me relax and sleep better but actually, all it did was overstimulate my adrenals and disturb my sleep. Alcohol also interferes with REM sleep which is vital to our having adequate rest and healing our adrenals. Also, when it comes to caffeine, it actually decreases the amount of melatonin (our sleep hormone) released by the pineal gland so that's another reason to cut the caffeine.

- **Don't exercise at night:** I'm going to be covering exercise next but you need to be cautious of what exercise you do and when, especially when it comes to your sleep. When you exercise later in the day it increases cortisol levels which can disrupt your sleep patterns. It's best to exercise in a morning when your energy levels are at their highest.

Exercise or Excess Insulin

Everyone tells you that exercise is good for you but, what if I told you that certain types of exercise are bad for you if you have insulin resistance?

Don't get too excited though, I'm not telling you that you shouldn't be exercising at all, I'm just saying you need to be cautious about the types of exercise that you should be doing.

How many times have you decided you are going to start an exercise regime only to push yourself too hard and give it up? You slog away for hours at the gym, you're working up a sweat in hour long spin classes or you seem to think you can go from zero to marathon training with no build up in-between. You feel like you're giving it your all but you're getting nowhere, instead you feel ready to burn out so throw in the towel and give up because it's not working for you.

Want to know a secret? Intense exercise like this is NOT going to help you, your blood sugar balance or your PMS, because all it does is put the body under stress and as we've discussed, cortisol and insulin have the ability to really spur each other along.

Pushing yourself to the limit will cause cortisol levels to rise and will cause your energy levels to flatline triggering the body to go into survival mode.

Now when you first start out with the exercise, everything seems fine and dandy, the body will initially use the energy from stores in the body which yay, is exactly what you wanted. But then, as energy levels dip, the body realises it needs to hold onto this energy so your body can carry out its vital functions and will actually increase the energy stores ... especially in the visceral fat which makes it almost impossible to lose weight (frustrating when this is why most of us exercise, right?).

In addition to that, the cortisol - insulin cycle and those decreased energy levels will increase your carbohydrate cravings which again can cause blood sugar spikes and release those inflammatory proteins that contribute to insulin resistance.

So what type of exercise should you do? If you are looking to balance blood sugars, then the best forms of exercise are:

- **HIIT workouts:** These can help consume excess sugars and improve insulin resistance.

- **Yoga:** This has been found to be beneficial for balancing blood sugars, decreasing stress levels and decreasing obesity levels (especially in diabetics).

- **Resistance Training:** Weight lifting in moderation ... remember, nothing too intense! This helps remove fat from the muscle which means the muscles can take up the glucose better.

Always be sure to choose a type of exercise that you enjoy, that way you are more likely to stick to it than if you are forcing yourself to do something you don't want to. As a hater of breaking a sweat and a self-confessed lazy gal, my personal favourites are walking the dogs, yoga and Pilates but I can be partial to a bit of belly dancing or swimming. Remember, do what you love, and love what you do.

Part 4: Vitamins & Minerals

How vitamins and mineral deficiencies impact on your PMS

Our bodies need a balance of over 50 vitamins and minerals, and although it's incredibly rare to be deficient in protein, fat or carbohydrates, vitamin and mineral deficiencies are incredibly common, with an estimated 9 out of 10 of us not receiving sufficient vitamins and minerals from our diet. No surprise, when you consider what todays 'traditional' diet is like.

However, a deficiency in any of these can impact on our hormones, especially vitamin B, vitamin D, zinc, calcium and magnesium which play a crucial role in hormone balance. There have been several studies carried out that have looked at the impact of these vitamin and mineral levels on the severity of PMS symptoms.

One of those studies, by Saeedian et al (2015), specifically looked at the roles of vitamin D, calcium and magnesium in relation to PMS. During their study, which consisted of 62 women, aged between 20 and 22 of which 31 of them were pre-diagnosed with PMS, they identified that subjects with PMS did show nutritional deficiencies in calcium, magnesium and vitamin D.

Levels of calcium and magnesium were also lower in those who did not have PMS, although the ranges in these women were still classed as being within 'normal' levels. In fact, during their study they actually discovered that a whopping 85% of the study participants had vitamin D deficiency and, that more than one third of the PMS subjects were deficient in magnesium.

But what roles do these vitamins play? I will be looking at each of these vitamins and minerals in closer detail but overall, essential fatty acids, vitamin B6, zinc and magnesium are all involved in the body creating prostaglandins which also help to balance hormones and keep those menstrual cramps at bay.

Prostaglandin is a hormone produced not throughout the body, but in the place it is required at the time, namely to help the body deal with injury or illness by helping fight inflammation. However, there is research to suggest that women with PMS have lower levels of production in the luteal phase (the phase right before your period) which means we aren't getting enough of the anti-inflammatory prostaglandins to tackle the pain and inflammation, hence those goddamn awful cramps.

These statistics just go to show how important a carefully balanced diet is when it comes to regaining control over your PMS hell. This section of the book will look at the main vitamins known to impact on PMS and look at ways you can address these through dietary changes.

However, if you feel like diet alone will not be sufficient and you want to consider supplementation then I am offering readers of my book a 50% discount off my personalised dietary supplementation plans. The plan will take you through a series of online lifestyle and dietary questionnaires, once completed I then personally develop you a fully personalised plan which includes the supplements you most need to take and the recommended dosages.

You can order your personalised supplementation plan on my website www.emmalouisekirkham.com, and don't forget to enter the code PMSHELL at the checkout to get your discount.

Essential Fatty Acids

We have been brainwashed for years that fats are bad, so much so that now the supermarket shelves are filled with an array of low-fat and fat-free products. Slimming groups encourage the use of these products so for those struggling with weight loss or thinking they are being 'healthy', low-fat and fat-free products have become a part of everyday life.

However, when we follow a low-fat diet we are often preventing ourselves from being able to digest fat-soluble vitamins such as vitamins A, E, D and K. These vitamins play a huge role in hormone balance and being unable to absorb them puts you at greater risk of vitamin deficiency.

Let's start by looking at what essential fatty acids are. Essential fatty acids are long chain fatty acids - these types of fatty acids are packaged and stored by the body for later use, and are harder for the body to burn. They are essential in order to achieve normal function but, as the body can't produce them by itself, they have to come from either diet or supplementation. The two essential fatty acids are Omega-3 (also known as alpha linolenic acid) and Omega-6 (also known as linoleic acid).

Both Omega-3 and Omega-6 have been shown to help alleviate PMS symptoms. A study by

Sohrabi et al. (2013) identified that Omega-3 fatty acids helped alleviate the psychological symptoms of PMS such as depression, anxiety and lack of concentration, and may also reduce issues such as bloating, headaches and breast tenderness. Other studies have also reported improvements in PMS symptoms when increasing intake of essential fatty acids, especially in the luteal period.

If you decide to go down the supplement route, it's worth knowing that one study also identified that women who took supplements for six months saw better benefits than those who only took the supplements for three months, which indicates that keeping taking those essential fatty acid supplements long term will be more beneficial when it comes to managing your PMS.

The optimal ratio of Omega-6 to Omega-3 is 4:1, however, with todays westernised diet, it's more like 20:1 which is why the majority of studies focus on Omega-3. However, both types of Omega provide their own benefits; Omega-3 is said to help reduce the symptoms of PMS and those pesky menstrual cramps while Omega-6 can help reduce the depression, irritability and headaches that are linked to PMS.

In addition to that, these essential fats can also help to balance all of our hormones, which can help achieve optimal ovulation and, in turn, improve fertility. They also help decrease inflammation in the body and can help us maintain an ideal body composition (as in it helps maintain a healthy weight).

Always make sure you are getting the best types of essential fatty acids into your diet as some fats such as rancid fats found in many processed foods (including roasted nuts) and trans fats in baked foods and fried foods actually have a negative impact on our bodies and our hormones as they increase inflammation in the body, disrupt our sex hormones and can disrupt our estrogen levels.

The best food sources for your essential fatty acids are:

- Wild caught fish such as salmon and sardines
- Grass-fed beef (grass fed cattle have higher levels of antioxidants and vitamins that are required for hormone balancing)
- Pasture raised eggs
- Full fat cheese and yogurt*
- Extra virgin olive oil
- Organic avocados
- Raw, soaked nuts and seeds
- Cold pressed, unrefined coconut oil
- Grass-fed butter*

*If you do have any allergies towards dairy, skip the cheese, yogurt and butter!

As part of regaining control over your PMS, try to add at least two of these into your day every day. Try having avocado and egg on wholemeal toast for breakfast, drizzle some olive oil over your salad or potatoes instead of adding butter at lunch or dinner, enjoy a piece of pan-fried salmon with crispy skin or, instead of a sweet dessert after a meal, enjoy some sliced apple and cheese. The possibilities are endless!

Vitamin B6

Vitamin B6, also known as pyridoxine, is well known for its role in hormone production. It helps to balance the sex hormones and help maintain optimal levels of progesterone, which is why its commonly acknowledged for its role in helping with PMS.

In addition to this, vitamin B6 is also a natural anti-depressant and diuretic which makes it good for the psychological symptoms of PMS and that pre-period water retention that has us piling on the pounds when we get weighed!

There have been numerous studies on the use of vitamin B6 for the treatment of PMS and the best dosages. One study by Wyatt et al. (1999) identified that 50mg vitamin B6 taken daily was beneficial for relieving PMS symptoms. Another study by Masoumi, Atollahi and Oshvandi (2016) identified the benefits of vitamin B6 on premenstrual symptoms was enhanced further when combined with calcium (which is a mineral we will also be looking at in this book).

We looked at excess estrogen earlier in the book, but just to remind you that vitamin B6 also helps the liver to break down excess estrogen so the body can remove it. If you have a B6 deficiency and the liver can't keep up with breaking down the excess estrogen, then this can increase estrogen levels in the body. It's like a vicious cycle isn't it (there she goes again with those vicious cycles!).

The best food sources for vitamin B6 are:

- Fish, such as salmon and tuna
- Beef liver and other organ meats
- Turkey
- Starchy vegetables and fruits, such as bananas, broccoli, cauliflower, peppers, and Brussel sprouts
- Pasture raised eggs
- Wheatgerm
- Red kidney beans

Great ways to get these into your diet could include a tuna and egg salad, salmon and Mediterranean vegetables, a turkey mince chilli with red kidney beans. Don't be afraid to get creative in that kitchen and experiment a little.

As a supplement, I'd personally recommend a B-Complex as the B vitamins as a whole play a crucial role in the regulation of the menstrual cycle and work very synergistically together. In addition, the B vitamins are easily depleted when you are stressed, so it's important to keep levels maintained, especially as we've already discussed how we tend to live in a constant state of stress.

Vitamin D

Vitamin D, often referred to as the sunshine vitamin, is well known for its role in calcium absorption and maintenance of calcium levels but it's also been studied extensively and found to help reduce PMS and those pesky menstrual cramps, as well as helping to regulate our immune system.

Vitamin D comes in two different forms; ergocalciferol (D2) which is found in some plant-based foods, and cholecalciferol (D3) which is found in mostly fish, meat and dairy. Many studies have identified that the D3 form is more effective at raising vitamin D levels in the blood.

D3 is the form of vitamin D that the body can create it on its own. The reason it's been called the sunshine drug is the common belief that just 15 minutes of daily sun exposure is enough for your skin to produce enough vitamin D. However, this is not necessarily the case as people do not tend to take into consideration cloud coverage, pollution levels in the sky, and the wearing of sunscreen, which is going to block those UV rays.

Something you may not know, is that vitamin D is also known as the period hormone, because it plays in important role in menstrual cycle regulation. It's been shown to have a positive impact on PCOS and endometriosis, and plays an important role in improving fertility.

During a review of 28 journal articles and written papers, Abdi, Ozgoli and Rahnemaie (2019) concluded that low levels of vitamin D (and calcium) during the luteal phase of the cycle caused or worsened the effects of PMS. They also noted that women whose diets were high in foods containing calcium and vitamin D were at a lower risk of developing PMS.

Interestingly, darker skinned individuals are less able to produce vitamin D than lighter skinned individuals, which is likely related to the increased melanin in their skin that protects from UV light.

Also, if you follow a vegan diet, you are also more likely to be deficient in vitamin D as it's not found in many vegan-friendly foods so you would benefit from supplementing this. In fact, it's worth noting that vitamin D is difficult to obtain from food alone, even if you're a meat eater.

When you consider that many of us do not get enough adequate sun exposure, and the fact it's so hard to get from our food supply, this shows the importance of having a balanced and nutrient packed diet when looking to tackle your PMS symptoms, and the benefits of supplementing with a D3 supplement.

The best food sources for vitamin D to include into your diet are:

- Fatty fish such as mackerel, salmon, tuna and herrings
- Eggs
- Cottage cheese and butter
- Mushrooms (that have been grown in UV light)

Zinc

Although this chapter is about vitamins and minerals, we also need to look at some of the trace elements, such as zinc, which can also be beneficial to women who suffer with PMS.

Zinc is involved in over 300 enzymatic activities in the body, playing an important role in immunity, gene regulation and a process called apoptosis (which is a natural cell death in the body).

When it comes to our hormones, Zinc has an influence on hormone release and nerve impulse transmission, supports healthy ovulation, helps to maintain and increase testosterone levels (which also helps keep that sex drive alive and raring to go!) and can support progesterone production.

Again, as with the other vitamins, zinc has been the subject of several studies which has looked at how it can help support women who suffer from PMS.

One of those studies, by Jafari et al. (2020), identified that 12 weeks supplementation of zinc was beneficial to the quality of life in women with PMS which reiterates what I said at the start of this book about supplements requiring a minimum of 12 weeks to show results. This is likely down to the fact that levels of zinc seem to drop during the luteal phase in women who suffer with PMS.

The need for zinc was also backed up in a study by Chuong and Dawson (1994) who discovered that women with PMS appeared to suffer with both zinc deficiency, as well as increased copper levels in their luteal phase of the menstrual cycle. They also noted that copper competed with zinc for intestinal absorption which is what made the zinc levels lower and less available for the body to use.

Increasing zinc levels in the run up to and during the luteal phase alongside controlling your stress, as stress can rapidly decrease zinc levels too, can therefore help prevent that deficiency which can, in turn, help alleviate some of those PMS symptoms. However, ladies, if you are on a vegan or plant-based diet then you may need to supplement this as very few plants contain zinc.

The best food sources for Zinc are:

- Oysters
- Shrimp
- Ginger root
- Lamb
- Dry Split Peas
- Nuts (especially Brazil Nuts, Pecans, Peanuts)
- Whole Wheat Grain and Rye
- Oats
- Egg Yolks

Now, let me tell you this ... Oysters, as well as being an aphrodisiac, are by far the HIGHEST source of zinc so if you're still in that honeymoon phase of your relationship or looking to reignite the 'romance' as your hormones have sent your sex drive packing, then indulging in this shellfish gives you a double whammy. You, and your partner, can thank me later for that little nugget!

Other ways to incorporate these foods into your diet could be a lamb tagine, a seafood platter, a prawn biriyani, or even making your own healthy flapjack with oats and added nuts.

Calcium

I don't know about you, but when I hear calcium I automatically think of dairy, or that its good for your bones, but how often do you think that calcium could play a role in your PMS symptoms? I bet you don't ... until now that is!

Yes, calcium is essential to our bones and teeth, it promotes a healthy heart and helps with blood clotting amongst other things, but when it comes to us ladies and our PMS, calcium plays an important role in the secretion of hormones, can reduce menstrual cramps and can help alleviate some of our PMS symptoms ... if we have adequate levels that is.

There have been several research papers that have looked at the impact of calcium levels on PMS and it has been noted in many of them that women who suffer with PMS do appear to have low levels of calcium.

One study by Shobeiri et al. (2017) looked at the effect on PMS of supplementing calcium over a two-month period. Although they saw little change in the first month, during the second month they observed that the calcium supplements gave a significant decrease in the mood-related symptoms of PMS, such as depression and sadness. This was shown to be more effective when supplementation was taken over a longer period of time and also when taken in conjunction with vitamin B6.

Arab et al. (2020) conducted a review of 14 different research papers that looked at the impact of calcium on PMS. During the review it was discovered, in the majority of the papers, that low levels of calcium were noted in women who suffered with PMS and, that calcium supplementation did indeed appear to help alleviate the symptoms of PMS.

When it comes to boosting calcium levels, it is always best to try to get it from food sources as the body can absorb it better this way. But, it's also worth noting that calcium absorption is improved further when combined with foods that also include vitamin D and magnesium. As such, many people who supplement this tend to supplement with a combined calcium and magnesium supplement (we will be looking at magnesium next).

The best food sources for Calcium are:

- Dark, leafy greens such as kale and spinach
- Full fat dairy products (organic is generally best) especially Swiss cheese and cheddar cheese
- Sweet Potatoes
- Sardines
- Almonds
- Brewer's Yeast

- Pumpkin seeds

Obviously if you are intolerant to dairy, then it best to avoid the cheeses! However, if you're not then here's your excuse for a cheese and crackers night but, be sure to avoid the wine as alcohol hinders the absorption of calcium (as well as many other vitamins and minerals). Sweet potato hashes are also a great way to use up any leftovers in the fridge and throw in all the vegetables you've got lying around (bonus points if they are veggies that are good for your PMS).

Magnesium

Magnesium is an incredibly important mineral for our health as, just like zinc, it plays a role in over 300 enzyme reactions in the body. It's involved in several functions including ion transportation, cell signaling and energy production.

An adult body contains around 25g magnesium, of which 50% - 60% of it is stored in our bones, which does help to explain why calcium and magnesium work so well when combined with each other. But, how does it help with your PMS?

Magnesium promotes healthy muscles and helps them to relax, which means it plays a major role in how bad those menstrual cramps are and, surprisingly, a deficiency in this mineral is incredibly common. Magnesium deficiency is actually a major contributing cause to women having bad menstrual cramps, as women with PMS tend to have lower levels of magnesium that women who do not suffer with it.

A study by Facchinetti et al. (1991) looked at supplementation of magnesium and its impact on PMS. The women who were given the supplements over the two-month trial reported a significant reduction in menstrual pain compared to those who were given the placebo.

And it's not just calcium that magnesium works well with either. A more recent study by Fathizadeh et. al (2010) determined that a combination of magnesium supplements with vitamin B6 supplements were more effective than just magnesium alone when addressing PMS. This makes absolute sense, as you are then tackling both the physical and the psychological issues of PMS.

So, as you can see, magnesium works especially well with combined with the other vitamins and minerals we've already discussed (B-vitamins, vitamin C, vitamin D, zinc and calcium) as they help promote the absorption of magnesium and will ultimately help tackle those pesky PMS symptoms.

The best food sources for Magnesium are:

- Seeds (pumpkin seeds, sesame seeds, flax seeds and sunflower seeds)
- Wheat germ
- Nuts (almonds, cashew nuts, Brazil nuts and pecans)
- Brewer's Yeast
- Dark, leafy greens
- Dark Chocolate

Yes, I said chocolate … so when the PMS chocolate cravings kick in, you CAN indulge provided you go for a high-quality dark chocolate. I'd recommend choosing a chocolate that is at least 80% cocoa as this isn't as full of sugar as a bar of

Dairy Milk or Galaxy is, and will contain vital antioxidants.

However, you do need to approach magnesium with care as it can be toxic at certain levels. If you are getting your magnesium from food, then toxicity is rare as the body metabolises it slower and any excess is passed out in the urine but, it can be toxic at levels over 1000mg. As such, care should be taken when supplementing and I'd always recommend getting advice from a professional (such as myself ... shameless plug there!).

Support your PMS with Nutrition

So now you've got the lowdown on the key vitamins and minerals that have an impact on, and can help improve your PMS. Has anything in here surprised you or were you already aware of the impact that nutrient deficiencies have?

I'd recommend spending the next week or two looking at ways to incorporate some of these foods into your diet. Aim to eat a wide variety of foods and aim to keep your plate colourful at each meal. You can plan out your meals in the downloadable workbook that works alongside this book, so if you haven't got it yet go grab yours from my website and be sure to use the code WORKBOOK to get 50% off.

Or, if you'd like to look at supplementing any of these nutrients and would like more advice, order your **Personalised Supplementation Plan** from me so I can ensure you are getting the right balance of vitamins and minerals in your diet based on your own specific requirements and symptoms. Don't forget you can also get 50% off your plan using the code PMSHELL at checkout.

Part 5: Moving into PMS Harmony

Keep Going

You did it! You've reached the end of the book but before you crack out the fizz to start the celebrations, your work doesn't end here ... the advice I've given you is for a lifetime, not just a quick fix.

As I mentioned right at the start, the journey from PMS Hell to PMS Harmony isn't instant. You'll need to really commit to following the advice given in here for at least three months, but if I'm honest ... you want to follow the advice forever as PMS won't just magically disappear and, as I mentioned earlier in the book, it's only going to get worse with age.

That's not to say you can't have a social life or a little overindulgence now and then. We all have days where we might have a cheeky chocolate fix, or we go out for drinks and dinner ... that's okay, and its often something as women we fail to accept.

You have to be gentle and forgiving with yourself.

Yep, I got all hippy towards the end didn't I and started giving you the self-love stuff ... but it's true. As women we are our worst critics. We punish ourselves unnecessarily and it's time for that to STOP!

I mean, let's face it, its counterproductive. It's going to increase your stress and probably cause you to binge eat and undo all the good work you've been doing … because so many of us are emotional eaters. If that isn't a good enough reason then I don't know what is.

We can achieve a hell of a lot alone, but together we can achieve so much more. Share your successes … share your journey (and feel free to tag me in your social media posts so I can see how you are getting on … its @emmalouisekirkham on both Instagram and YouTube.

I want to see and share your successes, I want to hear and help support you with your struggles, and I want to hear about your wins, no matter how big or small they may seem. So please, do check in with me to let me know how things are going.

Your journey isn't over yet … you're in a new phase. The transition from PMS Hell to PMS Harmony and I am so grateful you chose me to help you on the journey.

Much love

Emma x

Resources

I know what it's like keeping flicking through books to try and find that one page that contains a link or a resource so, to make your life easy, I've compiled everything here for you so that you've got a handy reference guide.

Menstrual Cycle Guide: This is my free guide that gives you hints and tips on the foods and activities that are best for each stage of your menstrual cycle. Get your free copy from https://mailchi.mp/3ed2953aafe7/menstrualguide

The PMS Hell to PMS Harmony Workbook: The workbook gives you space to plan out and track for 12 weeks, which is the minimum time I recommend following this advice for, so do be sure to get your copy. Another benefit of the workbook is that you have an easy reference to previous weeks plans, so if you had a particularly good week you can the replicate it. Get your workbook from https://emmalouisekirkham.com/product/pms-hell-to-pms-harmony-workbook/

As a reader of my book, I'm also offering 50% off the listed price, just enter the code WORKBOOK at checkout.

Personalised Supplementation Plans: Take the guesswork out of which supplements you should be taking and order your tailor-made plan from https://emmalouisekirkham.com/product/personalised-supplementation-plans/

Remember, I'm also offering you a 50% discount on this as a valued reader of my book. Enter the code PMSHELL at checkout to get your discount.

The Dirty Dozen: The 12 foods you should buy organic as the commercial ones tend to contain the most pesticides. View the list at https://www.ewg.org/foodnews/dirty-dozen.php

Need Additional Support?

I know it's not always easy to go it alone.

Whether it's a lack of support at home, or simply a lack of willpower ... I understand and I'm here to help. You'll have days or weeks where you are smashing it, and then suddenly you feel like you've run into a brick wall.

That's when you need that extra support. Sometimes you just need a little helping hand to guide you back on your way, or someone who will keep you focused and on track. That's why I wanted to make you aware of other ways I can help you on your journey so that you can really drive those results home.

One to One Coaching
Whilst this book offers generalised advice, one to one coaching allows us to work through the various areas of your life on a personalised basis. This means we dig deeper to find the root issues that cause your hormonal imbalance and find strategies for you to implement to tackle these specific areas. Sometimes your biggest blocks are internal ones that often you don't realise are blocking your until you start to do some soul searching that is.

Group Coaching
Why not join the PMS Hell to PMS Harmony Group coaching program where I'll personally be

supporting you over a 12-week period to cover the main areas associated to your PMS symptoms? We will be working through the suggestions in this book in a structured way, and you'll have the opportunity to ask questions as you go. Visit my website **www.emmalouisekirkham.com** to find out more about this opportunity.

And on a final note, if you enjoyed this book please help an author out and leave a review to share your views with others. Reviews are critical to an author's success and helps others know what to expect when buying this book.

You'd make this author a very happy one!

References

Arab, A., Rafie, N., Askari, G., & Taghiabadi, M. (2020). Beneficial Role of Calcium in Premenstrual Syndrome: A Systematic Review of Current Literature. *International journal of preventive medicine*, *11*, 156. https://doi.org/10.4103/ijpvm.IJPVM_243_19

Baker FC, Siboza F, Fuller A. Temperature regulation in women: Effects of the menstrual cycle. Temperature *(Austin)*. 2020 Mar 22;7(3):226-262. doi: 10.1080/23328940.2020.1735927. PMID: 33123618; PMCID: PMC7575238.

Chuong CJ, Dawson EB. Zinc and copper levels in premenstrual syndrome. Fertil Steril. 1994 Aug;62(2):313-20. doi: 10.1016/s0015-0282(16)56884-8. PMID: 8034078.

Facchinetti F, Borella P, Sances G, Fioroni L, Nappi RE, Genazzani AR. Oral magnesium successfully relieves premenstrual mood changes. Obstet Gynecol. 1991 Aug;78(2):177-81. PMID: 2067759.

Fathizadeh, N., Ebrahimi, E., Valiani, M., Tavakoli, N., & Yar, M. H. (2010). Evaluating the effect of magnesium and magnesium plus vitamin B6 supplement on the severity of premenstrual syndrome. *Iranian journal of nursing and midwifery research*, *15*(Suppl 1), 401–405.

Gold, E. B., Wells, C., & Rasor, M. O. (2016). The Association of Inflammation with Premenstrual

Symptoms. *Journal of women's health (2002)*, *25*(9), 865–874. https://doi.org/10.1089/jwh.2015.5529

Jafari F, Tarrahi MJ, Farhang A, Amani R. Effect of zinc supplementation on quality of life and sleep quality in young women with premenstrual syndrome: a randomized, double-blind, placebo-controlled trial. Arch Gynecol Obstet. 2020 Sep;302(3):657-664. doi: 10.1007/s00 404-020-05628-w. Epub 2020 Jun 8. PMID: 32514756.

Jehan, S., Auguste, E., Hussain, M., Pandi-Perumal, S. R., Brzezinski, A., Gupta, R., Attarian, H., Jean-Louis, G., & McFarlane, S. I. (2016). Sleep and Premenstrual Syndrome. *Journal of sleep medicine and disorders*, *3*(5), 1061.

Kautzky-Willer (2018) The Relationship of the Intestinal Microbiome and the Menstrual Cycle - ClinicalTrials.gov. (online 2022). https://clinicaltrials.gov/ct2/show/NCT03581201

Masoumi, S. Z., Ataollahi, M., & Oshvandi, K. (2016). Effect of Combined Use of Calcium and Vitamin B6 on Premenstrual Syndrome Symptoms: a Randomized Clinical Trial. *Journal of caring sciences*, *5*(1), 67–73. https://doi.org/10.15171/jcs.2016.007

Patisaul, H. B., & Jefferson, W. (2010). The pros and cons of phytoestrogens. *Frontiers in neuroendocrinology*, *31*(4), 400–419. https://doi.org/10.1016/j.yfrne.2010.03.003

Qiao, M., Sun, P., Wang, H., Wang, Y., Zhan, X., Liu, H., Wang, X., Li, X., Wang, X., Wu, J., &

Wang, F. (2017). Epidemiological Distribution and Subtype Analysis of Premenstrual Dysphoric Disorder Syndromes and Symptoms Based on TCM Theories. *BioMed research international, 2017*, 4595016. https://doi.org/10.1155/2017/4595016

Rocha Filho EA, Lima JC, Pinho Neto JS, Montarroyos U. Essential fatty acids for premenstrual syndrome and their effect on prolactin and total cholesterol levels: a randomized, double blind, placebo-controlled study. *Reprod Health.* 2011 Jan 17;8:2. doi: 10.1186/1742-4755-8-2. PMID: 21241460; PMCID: PMC3033240.

Roomruangwong, C., Carvalho, A., Geffard, M., & Maes, M. (2019). The menstrual cycle may not be limited to the endometrium but also may impact gut permeability. *Acta Neuropsychiatrica, 31*(6), 294-304. doi:10.1017/neu.2019.30

Saeedian Kia, A., Amani, R., & Cheraghian, B. (2015). The Association between the Risk of Premenstrual Syndrome and Vitamin D, Calcium, and Magnesium Status among University Students: A Case Control Study. *Health promotion perspectives*, 5(3), 225-230. Https://doi.org/10.15171/hpp.2015.027

Shimobayashi, Mitsugu, et al. "Insulin Resistance Causes Inflammation in Adipose Tissue." *The Journal of Clinical Investigation*, American Society for Clinical Investigation, 2 Apr. 2018, https://www.jci.org/articles/view/96139.
Shobeiri, F., Araste, F. E., Ebrahimi, R., Jenabi, E., & Nazari, M. (2017). Effect of calcium on premenstrual syndrome: A double-blind randomized

clinical trial. *Obstetrics & gynecology science*, *60*(1), 100–105.
https://doi.org/10.5468/ogs.2017.60.1.100

Sohrabi N, Kashanian M, Ghafoori SS, Malakouti SK. Evaluation of the effect of omega-3 fatty acids in the treatment of premenstrual syndrome: "a pilot trial". *Complement Ther Med*. 2013 Jun;21(3):141-6. doi: 10.1016/j.ctim.2012.12.008. Epub 2013 Jan 16. PMID: 23642943

Study: Fatty acids can help ease PMS symptoms. (2022). Retrieved 29 April 2022, from http://edition.cnn.com/2011/HEALTH/01/17/fatty.acids.pms/index.html

Weatherly, L. M., & Gosse, J. A. (2017). Triclosan exposure, transformation, and human health effects. *Journal of toxicology and environmental health. Part B, Critical reviews*, *20*(8), 447–469.
https://doi.org/10.1080/10937404.2017.1399306

Wyatt, K. M., Dimmock, P. W., Jones, P. W., & Shaughn O'Brien, P. M. (1999). Efficacy of vitamin B-6 in the treatment of premenstrual syndrome: systematic review. *BMJ (Clinical research ed.)*, *318*(7195), 1375–1381.
https://doi.org/10.1136/bmj.318.7195.1375

Zatterale, F., Longo, M., Naderi, J., Raciti, G. A., Desiderio, A., Miele, C., & Beguinot, F. (2020, January 29). *Chronic adipose tissue inflammation linking obesity to insulin resistance and type 2 diabetes*. Frontiers.
https://www.frontiersin.org/articles/10.3389/fphys.2019.01607/full

About the Author

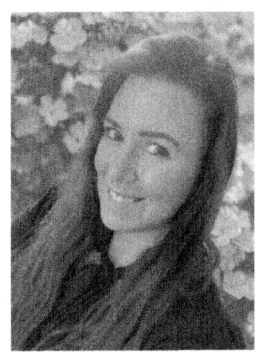

Emma Louise Kirkham is a health coach and dietary supplements advisor who specialises in women's hormone health.

Having trained with both the Institute of Integrative Nutrition and The Health Sciences Academy in many areas surrounding Nutrition and Coaching, as well as working in the body contouring industry as a therapist and educator since 2014, Emma has made it her mission to help women regain control over raging emotions and health issues associated to hormone imbalance.

Originally from Huddersfield, West Yorkshire, UK, Emma took a leap of faith and moved to the Algarve, Portugal in 2021 in order to restore harmony in her own life and regain control over her own hormonal issues as she hit her early 40's and even worse than before PMS.

Now, she's sharing with you the knowledge and experience she shares with her coaching clients in her debut book PMS Hell to PMS Harmony.

Find out more about Emma and her services by visiting her website: www.emmalouisekirkham.com

Or follow her on social media:

YouTube: https://www.youtube.com/@emmalouisekirkham
Instagram:
http://www.instagram.com/emmalouisekirkham
Facebook:
www.facebook.com/hormonehelltohormoneharmony

Printed in Great Britain
by Amazon